50 Days
of Hope

*Daily Inspiration
for Your Journey through Cancer*

Lynn Eib

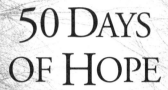

*The nonfiction imprint of
Tyndale House Publishers, Inc.*

Visit Tyndale online at www.tyndale.com.

Visit Tyndale Momentum online at www.tyndalemomentum.com.

Visit Lynn Eib's website at www.lynneib.com.

TYNDALE, *Tyndale Momentum*, and Tyndale's quill logo are registered trademarks of Tyndale House Publishers, Inc. The Tyndale Momentum logo is a trademark of Tyndale House Publishers, Inc. Tyndale Momentum is the nonfiction imprint of Tyndale House Publishers, Inc., Carol Stream, Illinois.

50 Days of Hope: Daily Inspiration for Your Journey through Cancer

For information about special discounts for bulk purchases, please contact Tyndale House Publishers at csresponse@tyndale.com, or call 1-800-323-9400.

Library of Congress Cataloging-in-Publication Data

Eib, Lynn.
    50 days of hope : daily inspiration for your journey through cancer / Lynn Eib.
        p. cm.
    Includes bibliographical references (p. 227-229).
    ISBN 978-1-4143-6449-0 (sc leatherlike)
    1. Cancer—Patients—Prayers and devotions. I. Title.
BV4910.33.E358 2012
242′.4—dc23   2011046237

Printed in China

23   22   21   20   19
11   10   9   8   7

This book is lovingly dedicated

in memory of my father

ROBERT YOXTHEIMER

1925–2011

a two-time cancer survivor,

and

in honor of my mother

GAYNOR YOXTHEIMER

a new cancer survivor

in 2011.

CONTENTS

APPENDIXES

ACKNOWLEDGMENTS

I am so grateful to:

- God for allowing me to survive cancer. I can't say I know exactly why He did, but I know I want to live my life in thankfulness to Him.

- My fabulous family for loving me and rejoicing with me for God's blessings in our lives: my husband, Ralph; my daughters, Danielle, Bethany, and Lindsey; my sons-in-law, Frank and Josh; and my new grandson, Bauer Jackson. (Someday you'll understand why Grandma wants to cry tears of joy every time she sees your beautiful face!)

- Marc and Elizabeth Hirsh, who first recognized God's call on my life to minister to cancer patients and gave me the unbelievable opportunity to live it out—without you, *none* of this would have happened.

- My brother, Jim, for loving me and praying for me. You're the only non-cancer-survivor in our family now—please *don't* join the club!

- All the cancer survivors and their families who allowed me to share their stories of hope with you. (I think my main "claim to fame" in life is that I have more friends with cancer than anyone else!)

- My Cancer Prayer Support Group members—who eats better, laughs louder, and experiences God's hope more than we do? Thanks for putting up with me and my dumb jokes.

- My Wise Women of Esther Group—Jodi, Kristin, Bev, Sue, Amanda, Dody, and Lorie—for praying me through the second-hardest year of my life. I never would have made it without your laughter therapy!

- The Knox Group of Tyndale House Publishers for continuing to ask me to write (in spite of my constant doubts that I can pen another book). Thanks especially to Bonne Steffen, my wise and excellent editor, and to Sharon Leavitt, senior communications manager, whose prayers and caring heart mean so much to me.

GOT HOPE?

Hope.

It may just be the best word in the English language. It has synonyms like *expectation*, *longing*, *desire*, *confidence*, *trust*, and *faith*. All of its antonyms can be rolled into one all-encompassing word: *hopelessness*.

We use it when we want to describe some of our deepest emotions, with phrases such as *our only hope*, *no other hope*, *false hopes,* and the saddest one of all—*no more hope*.

Hope can take so many different forms and meanings and even change from hour to hour, but I believe it is the one thing all cancer patients and their loved ones can agree they need—hope for today and especially hope for tomorrow.

Each week I usually meet five or six people newly diagnosed with cancer. That's because I work as a patient advocate in an oncology office where it's my job to offer emotional and spiritual support to cancer patients and their caregivers. Since 1996 I've met thousands of folks facing dreaded cancer diagnoses and scores more who have attended my Cancer Prayer

Support Group since its inception in 1991. And even though I'm a cancer survivor of twenty-plus years, I don't ever assume I know *exactly* how all these cancer patients feel. And I certainly wouldn't presume to know exactly how you and your loved ones are feeling right now.

But I do know what it feels like:

To hear my name and "cancer" in a sentence together.

To wait agonizingly long for test results.

To struggle over treatment decisions.

To watch toxic chemo drip into my veins.

To wonder if I'd see my children grow up.

And I know what it feels like to hope against hope that cancer would not have the last say in my life.

You're holding in your hand *50 Days of Hope*. This little book will take you through what many cancer survivors say are the darkest times—the first few months after a cancer diagnosis. Of course, you can read it to find hope at *any* time on your cancer journey, but it's especially written for those who recently have received a cancer diagnosis for themselves or someone they love. It's daily doses of inspiration that can be read in just a couple of minutes, because I know sometimes it's hard to concentrate and read when you're stressed about your health or the health of a loved one.

When I give someone a copy of my first book, *When*

God & Cancer Meet, I usually say something like, "If you need to, you can put this book aside for a while and pick it up later when you're ready to read it." I am confident that at just the right time, each person will read the book and experience the encouragement God wants to bring. People all over the world have told me that is exactly what happened to them.

Some of this book's inspiration is taken from that first book because I wanted to take those stories and encouraging truths and put them in an easily digestible format even for the most shell-shocked new patient or loved one. Some inspiration is taken from my other books, *Finding the Light in Cancer's Shadow* and *When God & Grief Meet*. And much of this book is filled with new, hopeful stories, as well as insights gained from my front-row seat watching God work in the lives of cancer patients and their caregivers.

So if I were handing you a copy of *this* book, I'd ask you to start reading it *today*—just one day at a time, just a few moments each day. It's kind of like eating a little snack just to keep up your strength until you feel like having a full meal.

Cancer can deplete us physically, and just as our bodies can get malnourished, our spirits can too. That's why you need to feed your spirit every day with truth that inspires you on your journey with cancer.

I love how author Max Lucado explains that what seems like a disaster to us may not be nearly so ominous from God's perspective:

> He views your life the way you view a movie after you've read the book. When something bad happens, you feel the air sucked out of the theater. Everyone else gasps at the crisis on the screen. Not you. Why? You've read the book. You know how the good guy gets out of the tight spot. God views your life with the same confidence. He's not only read your story . . . he wrote it.[1]

Please don't starve yourself of the hope you need—turn the page and find out what can happen in your life when God and cancer meet.

Lynn Eib

DAY 1
Been There, Done That

This is the kind of book I wish I could have read when I was diagnosed with locally advanced colon cancer in 1990. I was only thirty-six, and my daughters were eight, ten, and twelve. My husband's first wife had died from ALS—Lou Gehrig's disease—some twenty years earlier. I desperately needed hope and encouragement.

Don't get me wrong; many people tried to give me that. They said things like, "You'll get through this," or, "It'll be okay." But I wanted to yell back at them, "How do you know? You've never been through this!"

I had the sense that it made them feel better to tell me I was going to be all right, but it didn't do much for me.

The first person to really give me hope was a woman named Pat who came up to me after my first cancer support group meeting at the local hospital, put her arm around me, walked me to my car, and told me I would make it through my chemotherapy.

Do you know why I believed her? Not because she had years of medical training or decades of worldly wisdom. I believed her because she sported a brightly colored scarf on her head, still bald from chemotherapy. I recognized that she *knew* because she had been there.

Pat was the first cancer survivor I ever knew personally. Now my life is filled with cancer survivors because I've spent the intervening years both as a volunteer cancer support group facilitator and as an employed patient advocate in my oncologist's office.

I have held the hands of thousands of people with cancer, listened to the fears in their hearts, and seen what gave them hope. I know that cancer patients and their caregivers are longing for encouragement as they try to make sense of what might seem like senseless suffering. It is my prayer that this book will bring you that hope.

I don't know about you, but the words I most longed to hear after my cancer diagnosis were, "Oops, we made a mistake—you don't really have cancer after all!" Obviously, that retraction never came, and I had to face the reality that my nightmare was not going away any time soon.

If I couldn't hear that my cancer diagnosis was a "mistake," the next best thing would have been to meet someone who had been in my situation and survived.

I wanted to meet a young mom with Stage 3 colorectal cancer, who had about a 40-percent chance of surviving and did just that. But I didn't know anyone remotely like that at the time.

I now know thousands of cancer survivors, including many young moms and even those with far worse odds than mine who are alive and well. I wish you and I could meet face-to-face and you could tell me your story and I could tell you about someone I know who has walked in your shoes and is doing well. My Cancer Prayer Support Group (which is believed to be the longest-running such faith-based group in the country) has all kinds of amazing survivor stories. In fact, most of the people in my group have been told their cancer is not curable, yet they still are doing well, and many of them are cancer-free years later. We have people surviving melanoma, lymphoma, leukemia, and multiple myeloma, as well as adrenal gland, pancreatic, brain, liver, lung, stomach, breast, esophageal, fallopian tube, tonsil, cervical, colorectal, ovarian, peritoneal, prostate, bladder, tongue, thyroid, kidney, and even penile cancer (I didn't even know there was such a thing until I met a fifteen-year survivor!).

Whose story would give you hope?

Jutta, a Stage 3 pancreatic cancer survivor since 1999 and still cancer-free?

Jim, diagnosed with a recurrent brain tumor in 2006, but in complete remission?

Maureen, whose journey with breast cancer showed her that God really heard her prayers?

Anne, a small-cell lung cancer survivor given about a 10-percent chance of cure in 1994 and living cancer-free?

Sandy, diagnosed with incurable ovarian cancer, but beating cancer nonetheless?

I'll share all these true, hope-filled stories and many others throughout this book. It is my prayer that as you read them, you will experience God's peace and power and presence as never before. I pray that you will believe God can be trusted to meet your deepest needs because you can see His faithfulness in these people's lives.

* *You can believe their stories because they have been there.*

* *You can believe me because I have been there.*

* *You can believe God because He promises He will be there.*

I know we probably don't know one another and may never meet, but would you allow me the privilege of praying for you right now? (Just fill in your name as you read.)

Lord, I don't know what will give _____ hope . . . but You do. I know that You love _____ very much, and I am asking and believing that You will fill _____'s heart with a confident expectation that in spite of a cancer diagnosis, there is hope. Send Your healing touch wherever it is needed—body, mind, and spirit. Amen.

DAY 2
Sliding on Black Ice

Have you ever been driving down the road when all of a sudden you hit a patch of black ice? If you live in a climate that experiences true winter, you know exactly what I mean.

You're cruising along on bare pavement one minute and sliding down the road the next. You're on black ice—a covering of ice so thin that the dark pavement still shows through. If you apply the brakes, they do nothing to stop your vehicle. Instead, you just keep sliding, maybe even sideways, until you find something *bigger* than you to stop your slide!

When I was diagnosed with colon cancer, I felt as

if I had hit a huge patch of black ice. I had been going merrily along in life—happily married to my pastor-husband and enjoying our three young daughters. I loved my career as a newspaper reporter and even found time to exercise regularly at the local Y.

I consider myself an organized, well-prepared person . . . but I never saw the black ice of cancer ahead of me.

It took me so much by surprise that I couldn't even think how to react.

I tapped the brakes and nothing happened. I still had cancer.

I pressed a little harder on the brakes and found out the cancer had spread to my lymph nodes.

I slammed on the brakes only to learn that the odds I would survive were less than the odds I wouldn't.

I was sliding sideways, out of control, and it was the scariest time of my life. Thankfully, I didn't crash, but I did find something bigger than me to stop my slide.

Actually, Someone.

I slid right into the big, open arms of an all-knowing God, who assured me that He had seen the black ice coming. I prayed He would just make the black ice disappear so I could be carefree once again, but He didn't. So I continued riding on the thin layer of black ice through surgery and six months of weekly chemotherapy, which included having to endure a drug to which I was allergic.

As I was finishing treatment, I made the "mistake" of asking my oncologist, Dr. Marc Hirsh, what happens if the chemo doesn't work.

"If the cancer does comes back, it probably will come back within two years, and you will die very quickly," Marc told me as he explained I had one and only one shot at being cured because no effective treatment for recurrent colon cancer existed at that time.

So the black ice of cancer turned into a nasty shadow hanging over my head.

I tried various methods to get rid of cancer's shadow. I closed my eyes tightly: *I don't see any shadow.* But it was hard to go through a normal day with my eyes closed.

I got very busy. *The shadow won't be able to catch up with me.* But shadows are much faster than I realized.

I thought positively. *That's not a shadow. It's a big, happy, black balloon!* But it sure was dark under there.

I don't know exactly where you or your loved one is along your cancer journey. Maybe you've been blindsided fairly recently by the black ice of cancer. Maybe you're still slamming on the brakes, trying to believe it isn't so. Perhaps you're scared because you can't steer the way you want to go. Maybe you're waiting for the crash and are half afraid to open your eyes. Perhaps you feel the oppression of cancer's shadow wherever you go.

I don't care how big the cancer is, how small the cure odds are, how little time a doctor says you or your loved one has, I have a message for you in these next few weeks: God is bigger than cancer, His light is brighter than cancer's shadow, and there is always hope in Him.

Why am I discouraged?
  Why is my heart so sad?
I will put my hope in God!
  PSALM 42:5

When doubts filled my mind,
  your comfort gave me renewed hope and cheer.
  PSALM 94:19

I'd like to pray Psalm 10:17 for you today:

LORD, *You know the hopes of the helpless. Surely You will hear their cries and comfort them. Amen.*

DAY 3
Happy Endings Only

If this hasn't happened to you yet, I'm pretty sure it will.

Someone finds out you or your loved one has cancer and begins to tell you a story about a relative or friend of theirs who had a similar cancer. I'm sure it's an attempt to identify with what you're going through, but unfortunately, as the story unfolds, it's *not* what you really want to hear.

People used to come up and tell me gruesome stories about their neighbor who had the same kind of cancer I did and just "wasted away" or their grandmother who was "racked with pain." I hated hearing these stories, but at first I tried to be polite and listen.

Finally, I decided I could take it no longer, and when people started a cancer story, I would interrupt them, smile, and say, "Does this story have a happy ending? Because if it doesn't, I don't want to hear it."

That reply really stopped people in their tracks, and I didn't have to listen to any more hopeless cancer stories.

You may want to adopt my approach as well. Many patients tell me they have and that, surprisingly, it worked quite well, even though some folks' mouths dropped open at the shock of being asked to stop talking midsentence! Eventually, you may be fine to listen to any and all stories, but at first I think it's best to stick with the happy endings.

All the patients in our office know that when I start to tell them a story, they can relax because it's going to have a happy ending. Either the person got cured or went into remission or lived much longer than predicted. So relax as you read this book each day; it's filled with endless hope and not hopeless endings.

But I will be honest with you up front because I think you would want that. This is *not* a book of formulas that promise if you do this or don't do that, your prayers will be answered *just* the way you want them to be. I know such books exist because cancer patients and their families often want to talk with me when such a prayer formula doesn't work for them.

The truth is that some people get cured of cancer on this earth and some don't. I join you in hoping and praying for your cure, but I want to remind you that no matter what does or doesn't happen to your health or your loved one's, you do *not* have to be a *cancer victim*.

I hate that term. It somehow implies cancer is the victor. It wins; we lose. While we can do little to choose whether we get cancer, I believe we can do a lot to choose whether we are its victims. I don't just mean whether we live or die. I mean how cancer affects us in the deepest parts of who we are.

I urge you today, whether you are the cancer patient or the caregiver, not to choose to become a *victim* of cancer. Do not let this disease seem more powerful than it is. Do not let it fill your mind, steal your peace, invade your soul, or destroy your hope. It has no power to do those things unless you *allow* it to.

As you take this unwanted journey with cancer, I believe you are going to discover two things:

☀ *You are a lot stronger than you think, and God is a lot greater than you think.*

If you had told me prior to June 1990 that I was going to be diagnosed with cancer and have to endure major surgery and six months of weekly chemo, I would have said, "There's no way I can face that." If you had a crystal ball and showed me the terrible side effects I would suffer because I was allergic to the main chemo drug and no alternative existed at that time, I would have said, "I can't do it." If you told me I would have to live with the knowledge that if my cancer came back, there was no second chance at a cure and I would die very quickly, I would have told you, "There's no way I can live like that."

But that's because I didn't have a true appreciation for how great God really is. Oh, I'd believed in Him and even served Him faithfully for many years, but until I suffered personally, I'd never experienced how powerful He really is. Now I've seen firsthand the amazing strength of the human spirit and the incomparable greatness of the Almighty God.

> *The LORD is good,*
> *a strong refuge when trouble comes.*
> *He is close to those who trust in him.*
> NAHUM 1:7

If you don't want to be defeated by cancer—no matter what it does or has done to you or your loved one—you need a supernatural touch from God.

May I pray for you?

Heavenly Father, cancer feels very big right now. Please show Your power in my new friend's life and let him/her see that this disease is very small and weak compared to Your amazing strength. Help him/her to choose not to be a victim. Amen.

DAY 4
Feelings vs. Facts

As we walk these fifty days together, I hope you'll see how many people share the strong emotions you may have felt after a cancer diagnosis. And while I can appreciate the popular psychology that feelings are "neither right nor wrong," I also know that feelings do *not* necessarily mirror the facts.

I witnessed this firsthand a few years ago when my husband and I headed out with my boss, Marc, and his wife, Elizabeth, for our annual Labor Day weekend cruise on their thirty-two-foot Bayliner. The weather looked rather foul, but Elizabeth had checked with her brother who lives right on the Gunpowder River leading into the Chesapeake Bay, and he assured us the weather reports didn't look that bad despite a hurricane that was heading northward up the coast. (We later learned he had accidentally listened to the *wrong* forecast.)

So we took off anyway, knowing that Marc and Elizabeth were seasoned boaters—although the whitecaps on the usually calm river should have been our first clue it wasn't a good idea.

We had a short two-hour cruise ahead of us, but it wasn't long before the whitecaps turned into three-foot waves. The wind whipped up, and then the thunder, lightning, and rain came. At first we all laughed and enjoyed the warm rain soaking us as the boat pounded through the waves. But then I stopped laughing and my stomach started rebelling. Elizabeth handed me a supply of Ziploc plastic bags, which I started filling.

The waves were now five feet high and crashing clear over the top of the boat's windshield, drenching us. It was nearly impossible for Marc to see through the rain-splattered windshield, and my husband and Elizabeth were trying to read the navigational charts and look for the numbered buoys, which would keep us in the correct channel away from large shipping vessels, shallow water, and crab pots. We were too far out to turn back toward home, yet not sure we could make it to our planned destination.

And then it got really bad.

Marc announced that according to the boat's compass, we were headed in exactly the wrong direction—south when we should have been heading north.

We all were sure we hadn't turned around—Elizabeth was especially positive we were still pointing in the right direction. She was convinced she would have noticed if the boat had made an about-face. From past experience I knew that she was usually right whenever the two of them had a boating disagreement.

The three of us looked at Marc, waiting to see what he would do. (Well, I didn't look long because I was busy praying there were enough Ziploc bags.)

After a long pause, Marc posed his now-famous question: "Should I trust my wife . . . or the magnetic poles of the earth?"

It wouldn't have surprised me if he'd gone with Elizabeth's feelings because she was so adamant about them, but his scientific brain won out, and Marc turned the boat 180 degrees.

Within a few moments, we sighted buoys, which confirmed that we indeed had been going in the wrong direction despite all of us "feeling" otherwise.

The storm raging around us had distorted reality, and our feelings had fallen fickle.

The same thing can happen in the storms of cancer. We can *feel* as if we're unable to cope or that we have no hope. These are the times we need a compass—something that always will steer us in the right direction. Don't worry; I'm not suggesting that I'll be that compass.

The God of the universe has a special affinity for

brokenhearted people, and His words are the perfect compass for people facing cancer. A magnetic compass always will point you to the North Pole, and God's Word *always* will point you to His unchanging truth and promises.

> *I weep with sorrow;*
> *encourage me by your word.*
> PSALM 119:28

I can't change the reality of the diagnosis you're facing. But I hope to show you or perhaps remind you that a deeper spiritual reality transcends our earthly reality. If you already think of the Bible as your guide to life, I know you'll appreciate these tender reminders. But if you've not seriously given God's Word central importance in your life, I hope you'll give it a try now. You really have nothing to lose and everything to gain.

> *I cry out for help and put my hope in your words.*
> PSALM 119:147

Like Marc as he captained our boat on that stormy trip, it's your choice whether or not to trust the magnetic poles of the earth. You might want to pray this prayer:

Father, I feel a little lost right now. Please guide me in all the decisions to be made, and help me to trust Your truth more than my feelings. Amen.

DAY 5
All Shook Up

It's amazing how quickly your world can fall apart. One minute life seems pretty good, and the next minute you're wondering how you ever will survive. On a big scale, events like the attack on Pearl Harbor, President Kennedy's assassination, and 9/11 remind us that life is precarious. (On a much smaller scale, one minute you're laughing in the summer rain on a boat ride, and the next minute you're losing your lunch into a plastic bag!)

A health crisis has the ability to shake our world in ways difficult to comprehend. Recently I surveyed a bunch of my cancer survivor friends for remembrances of the day their world fell apart.

Surreal is the term Wayne uses to describe how it felt to be told he had Stage 4 non-Hodgkin's lymphoma at the age of forty-seven.

"My family, like me, was in shock—pure disbelief,"

he recalls thirteen years later. "I recently had gone twenty years without missing a full day of work to illness, and now I had cancer? I couldn't believe it."

Ken was equally surprised nine years ago when his tongue cancer finally was diagnosed after two years of reassurances that the enlarged lymph node was "nothing to worry about."

"When the doctor finally did say the word *cancer*, I was in total shock," Ken recalls. "I had no symptoms, and I was in great shape for a forty-six-year-old man! I told someone I felt as if I had entered the Twilight Zone and nothing was recognizable."

Cathy says "denial and total shock" were the first two emotions she experienced after being told in November 2009 that she had breast cancer at age fifty-four.

"My husband's and my emotions were very different," she adds. "He was a lot calmer and stronger than I was."

My nurse/reporter friend Cubby says disbelief was her first reaction to a breast cancer diagnosis at age fifty-one.

"I froze and my husband's face turned white," she still vividly recalls six years later. "The worst part was the fear of the unknown."

☀ *Fear of the unknown.*

I think that's pretty much a universal response to a cancer diagnosis. The story of the day *your* world fell apart may be similar to these folks', or it might be quite different, but I'm willing to bet that after those initial strong emotions wore off, you were left with the same question for yourself or your loved one: What's going to happen next?

How difficult will the treatment be?

Will I/they get sick?

Can I/they keep working?

And the million-dollar question: Will I/they be cured?

I, of course, will answer all those questions for you in this book . . . yeah, right. I have no magic tea leaves for your or your loved one's future. I believe there's a good chance that the treatments will be easier than you think because that's what most of our patients say—the worry *before* the first chemo or radiation treatment was worse than the treatment itself. I think you or your loved one probably will *not* get sick because there are wonderful anti-nausea drugs available today—at least three or four new ones since I was treated in 1990. (If you know people treated a long time ago for cancer, please don't imagine your experience is likely to be the same.)

I also think there's a good possibility you or your loved one will be able to keep up a fairly normal life.

I see cancer patients every day in our office getting chemo and then heading out to their place of employment or home to do yard work. Most folks say they adjust to a "new normal" and enjoy the days with good energy, resting more on the days when fatigue sets in.

And if you want to know the overall survival odds, 66 percent of adult cancer patients are still alive five years after their diagnosis, according to the National Cancer Institute.[2]

Of course, I can't *promise* my observations will come true for you. I don't know your future health any more than I am certain of my own. But I do know the One who knows it all.

> *"For I know the plans I have for you," says the LORD. "They are plans for good and not for disaster, to give you a future and a hope."*
> JEREMIAH 29:11

What an incredibly comforting verse for us when our world falls apart. Just don't miss that itty-bitty word *I* in the first sentence. "For *I* know the plans *I* have for you."

Only God knows the plans for us and they are *His* plans, not necessarily ours. But whether His plans match ours or not, we can be confident they are good ones and designed to give us hope. Jeremiah 29:12-14 continues with God's assurances:

> *In those days when you pray, I will listen. If you look for me wholeheartedly, you will find me. I will be found by you.*

Thank You, Lord, that You are not watching me from a distance, but You are close by and hear me when I pray. Please help me to trust that Your plans for my life are truly good ones. Amen.

DAY 6
An Unwelcome Intruder

I don't know if this cancer diagnosis is the first one your family has faced or simply the latest in a string of bad health news. Lucky me . . . I was the first in our large extended family to find out my DNA had "slipped up" and allowed cancer to "slip in." At the time, I had plenty of relatives with diabetes and heart problems, but always thought cancer wasn't something lurking in our genes.

So while some folks might suspect they may get

a cancer diagnosis someday, I never did. Instead it seemed as if my cancer just came out of *nowhere* and struck when I least expected it. I hear many cancer patients say the same thing—some of them are even in their seventies and eighties but have enjoyed such good health that they felt immune to cancer.

And then there are those I meet who already have had cancer knocking at their family's door too many times—they've watched parents, spouses, grandparents, or even their children wage cancer battles and now are discouraged that it's their "turn."

I think it's hard to be the first in your family with cancer, and it's hard to be the latest one diagnosed. Either way, this disease is a very unwelcome intruder.

I know that's how my friend Guy felt when he was diagnosed in December 1993 with what his surgeon later would describe as "Stage D" prostate cancer (and yes, this story has a happy ending!).

In 1991, Peg, Guy's wife of thirty-four years, died from a rare, inoperable cancer, and his middle son, Mike, endured chemo and radiation for testicular cancer in 1992.

Now it was Guy's turn.

"I didn't get angry," he recalls, "but I felt very empty, and I said, 'Why, Lord, why?'"

Even though Guy had a strong faith in God before his diagnosis, it wasn't easy for him to face cancer without Peg at his side. But he was about to find out that this unwelcome intruder was no match for the Creator of the universe.

A radical prostatectomy was scheduled for late January 1994, and Guy remembers the anxious moments before he went under the surgeon's knife.

"Before I went into the OR, they prepped me, and Mike's minister was up to see me and asked if he could pray with me," Guy says. "Then they took me out of the room and down the hall.

"Before we got to the [operating room] door, I said, 'Stop!'" Guy recalls. "The guy pushing me said, 'What's wrong?' but I just told him again to stop.

"I looked up and pointed up and said, 'Lord, You know me and I know You—do with me what You will.' Once I said those words, I was so at peace, and I said to the guy who was pushing me, 'Let's go!'

"I left my cancer prognosis up to God, and I wasn't afraid of anything. I had a peace that I can't really describe."

I would describe what happened that moment as a close encounter of the *divine* kind.

As Guy reached out to God, he said a simple prayer of surrender, giving the Master of the universe permission to have His way in Guy's life. He did what I believe we all need to do: agree to let God simply be God.

☀ Let Him be the unfalteringly faithful God, willing to strengthen us for any and every circumstance.

☀ Let Him be the absolute sovereign God, wise enough to know how and when to answer any and every prayer.

☀ Let Him be the mighty, awesome God that He is, powerful enough to heal us at any and every level—powerful enough to heal my friend Guy—body, mind, and spirit.

Have you ever had a divine encounter with the Lord? If you have, you're probably already praying for another such special moment. But if you haven't, you may be a little wary (maybe even a *lot* wary!). I don't think you have anything to lose—and you have a great deal to gain—by reaching out to God and saying a simple prayer surrendering your situation to Him. You could pray something like this:

Dear God, You know me and I want to know You more.
I surrender this cancer to You and ask You to have Your way
in my/my loved one's life. I pray this in Jesus' name. Amen.

P.S. If you want more of the happy ending to Guy's story, you should know the surgery (which did *not* remove all the cancer) was followed by radiation and hormone treatments, and seventeen years later Guy, now in his eighties, continues to be entirely cancer-free. He usually can be found spreading cheer as he volunteers helping the "old folks" at a local nursing home.

DAY 7
The Fear Factor

Sometimes things move very quickly once you get a cancer diagnosis. I guess that's good, because you don't have much time to think about it. But it also makes life feel a little like a surreal, out-of-body experience: *Can that really be* me *everyone is talking about?*

My cancer was discovered on a Tuesday, and in less than a week I saw the surgeon, had blood taken, got a chest X-ray, "cleaned out" my colon (again!), and had the tumor removed.

Three days later, at 7 a.m., the surgeon and his resi-
dent delivered the pathology report as I lay alone in my
room. I could tell from their body language that the
news wasn't good. They stood against the wall at the
end of my hospital bed, as far away from me as they
could get and still be in the same room.

"Cancer was found in five of twenty lymph nodes,"
the surgeon explained matter-of-factly. "You will need
chemotherapy and radiation."

I began to cry, but no one moved to comfort me.

"Have you ever known anyone who underwent
chemotherapy?" he asked, seeming to grasp for words
to continue the conversation.

I nodded, recalling the two people I had known—
both of whom had died! I started hyperventilating.

Still, neither doctor moved toward me, but instead
the surgeon called a nurse to help me breathe into a
paper bag. How I wished the doctor had at least held
my hand for a moment or just patted my shoulder
and told me that this was not an automatic death
sentence.

"Do you want me to call your husband?" the
surgeon asked, still at the foot of my bed. I nodded
between sobbing gasps into my little brown bag.

Now I was really frightened. I desperately needed
Ralph. But for whatever reason, the surgeon did not

call him. So for three hours I lay in the room thinking about what it was going to be like to have chemotherapy pour through my veins. I had a little conversation with myself as I tried to control my weeping.

Get a grip on yourself, my head told my heart. *What are you so afraid of? Nausea and vomiting? You were sick night and day for six months with all three of your pregnancies. Mouth sores? You've had them before. Needles? You're not afraid of them. Losing your hair? It'll grow back. Don't be so vain,* my head attempted to calm me. But my heart didn't buy it. I just cried harder as I stroked the waist-length hair that I desperately wanted to keep.

Yes, that's what I'm afraid of, I admitted. *I don't want to look sick for my children and my husband. I can't imagine watching my hair fall out.* I disliked the vanity of my feelings, but it was how I felt.

I finally called Ralph at 10 a.m. I was shaking so badly my voice was barely audible, and he kept asking me to repeat everything.

"It's bad," I told him. "I need you right away."

I couldn't even get my lips to form the word *chemotherapy.* For me, the fear of facing that was worse than the initial shock of cancer.

Ralph arrived shortly. At about noon the surgeon strolled in and said he had just tried to call my husband but there was no answer. "By the way," he added, "did I mention that you won't lose your hair with the chemo?"

I didn't know whether to smack him or hug him.

My surgeon obviously did a good job operating on me as I'm still alive and well, but his bedside manner wouldn't have earned such a high grade. It was impersonal and rather unprofessional not to call my husband for almost five hours. I don't think I should have gotten that bad news all by myself or been left alone for all that time afterward.

But God used that doctor's "mistake" to draw me closer to Himself and to help me face my deepest fears. As I named my fears, they did not disappear, but they lost some of their power over me, and I began to find the courage to face them.

☀ *It definitely takes courage to face cancer, but courage is not living without fear—it's living despite the fear.*

I love the late psychiatrist M. Scott Peck's thoughts on the subject:

The absence of fear is not courage; the absence
of fear is some kind of brain damage. Courage
is the capacity to go ahead in spite of the fear,
or in spite of the pain.[3]

God will give you the courage you need to face your
fears and to live with the uncertainties cancer brings.
Jesus said,

> *These things I have spoken to you, so that in*
> *Me you may have peace. In the world you have*
> *tribulation, but take courage; I have overcome*
> *the world.*
> JOHN 16:33, NASB

If you'd like more verses to help you "fear not,"
please turn to page 207 for some of my favorites.

I hope Psalm 27:1, 3 can be your prayer today:

> *The LORD is my light and my salvation—so why should*
> *I be afraid? . . . Though a mighty army surrounds me, my*
> *heart will not be afraid. Even if I am attacked, I will remain*
> *confident. Amen.*

DAY 8
It's a Family Affair

We have a saying in our oncology office: when one person in a family has cancer, it's as if the whole family has cancer.

This cancer diagnosis will permeate your home and affect everyone who lives there and those closest to you, wherever they live. And if you have children in your home, the ripple effect may be especially pronounced.

I remember feeling really guilty that my diagnosis was making everyone so sad. I could hardly stand the pained look on my mother's face as she watched me, her firstborn, having to deal with such a precarious prognosis. And my poor husband . . . I felt terrible for him. He already had watched his first wife die a slow, debilitating death from Lou Gehrig's disease when she was just twenty-three. My diagnosis was his worst nightmare revisited.

Every time we got bad news and every time he had to take care of something for me, I said, "I'm sorry." It upset me terribly that what was happening to me filled him with worry and piled on extra work because I was too ill to take care of the house and the girls the way I normally did. So I kept apologizing.

I apologized so much that he firmly told me one day, "You keep saying you're sorry—don't do that anymore." To which I automatically replied, "I'm sorry."

I honestly feel that many days it was harder for my husband to be the one *without* cancer than it was for me to be the one *with* cancer. At least I could feel I was *doing* something to fight the cancer as I watched chemo drip into my veins or popped chemo pills into my mouth. My husband, like many caregivers, often felt he was helplessly standing by, unable to *do* anything about my situation.

As I meet with newly diagnosed patients in my office each week, I often can sense that the patient is handling the diagnosis better than the spouse or adult children are.

One friend diagnosed with cancer in her early sixties told me that her husband literally ran out of the room when the doctor told them it was cancer.

"His mother died of cancer, and I know it was really hard for him," my friend explains. "When he came back in the room, he never said a word about it."

Sometimes patients are in such a fog they don't

really respond much to the initial diagnosis, but family members feel its weight fully.

My journalist friend Mike says his wife's reaction to his colon cancer diagnosis at age thirty-five was very different from his.

"She was scared and upset; I was calm and reserved because I had no idea of the impending doom," Mike recalls. "The night of the diagnosis we argued because she didn't understand why I wasn't more upset and I didn't understand why she was so upset. It was a really difficult time for both of us."

Mike's experience is not at all unusual. We tend to marry our "opposites," and when it comes time to deal with a cancer diagnosis, we often have opposite ways of handling the situation. Often one partner "feels" more and the other "thinks" more.

My friend Ken, diagnosed with tongue cancer in 2002, says he and his wife had similar initial responses, but then "she took a different approach to the shocking news."

"I wanted to curl up in a ball and pretend it was a huge mistake," Ken recalls. "She wanted to know everything she could about the disease and the treatments available, so she went on the Internet, made phone calls, and did research."

It has been my observation after meeting literally thousands of newly diagnosed cancer patients that people tend to cope with cancer the same way they cope with life, and there's not a lot other family members can do to change that. And while there certainly are healthy and unhealthy ways of coping, there isn't just *one* right way to cope with a cancer diagnosis. Just because someone in your family sees things differently doesn't mean necessarily that one of you is wrong and one is right.

Thank God today for the people He has placed in your life to help you with your cancer journey. It's important that even though each of you has a different personality and coping style, you come together as one in your cancer journey. Remember, your fight is against cancer . . . not each other.

So my prayer for you today is from Ephesians 4:31-32:

Get rid of all bitterness, rage, anger, harsh words, and slander, as well as all types of evil behavior. Instead, be kind to each other, tenderhearted, forgiving one another, just as God through Christ has forgiven you. In the name of Jesus. Amen.

DAY 9
Ticked Off

If you had asked me after my diagnosis whether I was angry about my situation, I would have responded that I was not. After all, it's not really proper for a minister's wife to get angry, is it?

Well, let me share a couple of the things I thought and felt those first few days after my diagnosis, and you tell me what you think my state of mind might have been.

When I was in the hospital after my cancer surgery, a friend came into my room and told me God was going to teach me great things through this trial. I wanted to take the IV out of my arm, stab it in hers, and tell her, "*You* get in the bed and learn great things from God, because I don't want to learn this way."

Of course, I didn't actually say that to her. Instead I just smiled and hoped she would leave very soon.

A couple of days later I was waiting for the pathology report to see if my cancer had been caught early and cured or whether it was advanced and I would need chemotherapy and perhaps radiation. Lying in that bed, I had lots of time to talk with God.

"You are making a really big mistake here," I fumed. "There's absolutely nothing You can ever do to make up for this because it is too awful. And don't think You are going to pull me through this somehow and I'm going to go and minister to cancer patients, because I won't do it!"

Perhaps a wee bit of anger there?

When I look back on those early days after my diagnosis, I am incredulous at some of the things I thought and felt. But I was in such a state of shock and disbelief myself that I really was struggling to cope. At one point, I was so distraught that I told my husband, "I guess God really doesn't love me."

I don't remember saying it and find it hard to believe I was actually that despondent, but I know my husband isn't making things up.

So as I look back on those dark days after my diagnosis, I realize I experienced a bevy of emotions: shock, disbelief, denial, disappointment, frustration, sadness, worry, and, yes, anger.

I didn't have anyone at the time whom I felt comfortable "burdening" with my anger, so I just kept taking it to God. The Bible says He can read our minds (Psalm 139:1-4), so I figured I might as well just say all the awful things I was thinking and feeling because He knew them anyway.

Maybe you're not as angry as I was; perhaps you're only a little ticked. Then again, maybe "rage" better describes what you're feeling today.

Where can you go to dump it?

I suggest you run where all of us with great suffering need to run: to the only One whose shoulders are broad enough, whose arms are strong enough, and whose love is deep enough.

"It's all right—questions, pain, and stabbing anger can be poured out to the Infinite One and He will not be damaged. . . . For we beat on His chest from within the circle of His arms," writes author Susan Lenzkes.[4]

Can you visualize that for yourself—you crying out to God, beating your clenched fists upon His chest, while He is holding you in His loving arms?

I am exhausted from crying for help;
   my throat is parched.
My eyes are swollen with weeping,
   waiting for my God to help me.
   PSALM 69:3

My God, my God, why have you abandoned me?
   Why are you so far away when I groan for help?
Every day I call to you, my God, but you do not
    answer.
   Every night you hear my voice, but I find
    no relief.
   PSALM 22:1-2

And then after you've hurled your questions heavenward, don't forget to go to God's Word to find His response. A good place to start might be the promise He gave to Jeremiah, who was filled with so much grief he has been called "the weeping prophet":

> *I have loved you with an everlasting love;*
>   *I have drawn you with unfailing kindness.*
> *I will build you up again,*
>   *and you . . . will be rebuilt.*
> JEREMIAH 31:3-4, NIV

☀ *I believe God is the best place to turn to with your suffering. He'll either give you the answers you seek or the peace you need to live with the questions.*

My reporter friend Cubby fought against a range of emotions accompanied by many tears when she battled breast cancer. But she says she always found hope "when I could visualize Jesus sitting next to me or holding me safely nestled in His lap."

It was in those moments that the peace came to live with the unanswered questions.

Perhaps you would like to pray today with the psalmist (Psalm 61:1-3):

O God, listen to my cry! Hear my prayer! From the ends of the earth, I cry to you for help when my heart is over- whelmed. Lead me to the towering rock of safety, for you are my safe refuge. Amen.

DAY 10
Cancer, Blah, Blah, Blah

So, how are you doing with learning your new cancer vocabulary?

Tumor markers. Monoclonal antibodies. Angio-genesis inhibitors. Stereotactic radiation. Mediport. Neutropenia. Micrometastases.

Or how about the alphabet soup of acronyms?

CEA, PSA, KRAS, ER/PR, HER2/neu, VEGF, and BRCA, just to name a few.

Yikes! Someone please get me an interpreter, or at least a dictionary! (Never mind the dictionary—I just hit spell-check on my computer, and it didn't recognize most of the words in the second paragraph!)

I remember after my diagnosis I felt thrown into a whole new world I hadn't even known existed, and I would have been just as happy to stay oblivious about it! So many terms and phrases were tossed around, and basically all I heard was, "You need chemo and radiation, blah, blah, blah, blah, blah."

But after a while I was forced to stick my head out of my shell and start to learn this foreign language. I discovered my colon cancer was classified back then as Duke's C2, meaning it had spread locally to more than three lymph nodes. I found out that 5-Fu was short for fluorouracil, a chemo drug that had been around for many years, and no one in Marc's practice but me had been allergic to it.

By the time I started working for Marc six years after my diagnosis, I had mastered a few of the oncology terms, but was still in for a real education as I worked for the first time in a medical office. I constantly had to ask the nurses for explanations of medical jargon I heard: "What's a DVT? I thought he had a blood clot?"

"He does. *DVT* stands for 'deep vein thrombosis.'"

Why not BC for blood clot?

One day I noticed the nurse, Ruth, had written the initials SOB next to a patient's name on the daily schedule. I was curious why she would make such a disparaging remark about the gentleman—he didn't seem that cranky to me.

Afterward I asked her, and when she stopped laughing, she explained that "SOB" stood for "short of breath"!

My opinion is that doctors and nurses aren't all that

much smarter than the rest of us—they just have their own special foreign language so we patients don't feel as bright! (To all my doctor and nurse readers—that was a joke!)

Anyway, I've spent the last fifteen-plus years learning medical terms and especially oncology phrases so I can throw them around the dinner table with my husband: "We thought there was nothing we could do for the patient, but the immunohistochemistry showed KIT-positive and it's a GIST and we can use a tyrosine kinase inhibitor! Isn't that great news?"

My husband could barely contain his excitement as he asked me to pass the salt.

Even though I may have gone a little overboard with learning the medical language, I have been amazed to learn about the human body's intricacies. Our bodies are so complex that, in some ways, I'm not as surprised they break down, but am *more* surprised that they don't break down more often!

The Human Genome Project, completed in 2003, identified the twenty-thousand-plus genes in the human body and sequenced the three billion chemical base pairs that comprise our DNA, or hereditary code of life. Dr. Francis Collins, the head of the project, explains that the DNA in each human is "3 billion letters long, and written in a strange and cryptographic four-letter code."[5] The code is so complex, Collins says, that if someone were to read it out loud at three letters per second, it would take thirty-seven years.

You made all the delicate, inner parts of my body
*   and knit me together in my mother's womb.*
Thank you for making me so wonderfully complex!
*   Your workmanship is marvelous—how well*
*   I know it.*
PSALM 139:13-14

Even though Collins is one of the world's leading scientists, he is also a man of Christian faith who calls our DNA "the language of God."

"We have caught the first glimpse of our own instruction book, previously known only to God,"[6] Collins said when the Human Genome Project's completion was announced.

He later wrote, "Science is not threatened by God; it is enhanced. God is most certainly not threatened by science; He made it all possible."[7]

You watched me as I was being formed in utter
*   seclusion,*
*   as I was woven together in the dark of the womb.*
PSALM 139:15

So just maybe the next time you hear some multi-syllabic medical words that seem overwhelming, you can allow them to remind you that you are "fearfully and wonderfully made" by the Creator of the universe and that your tomorrows are safe in His hands.

You saw me before I was born.
   Every day of my life was recorded in your book.
Every moment was laid out
   before a single day had passed.
   PSALM 139:16

Lord, thank You for doctors and nurses and researchers who are trying to cure cancer. I ask today that Your super-natural healing power would be released to heal the cancer in each cell that You created. In Jesus' name. Amen.

DAY 11
That's Not Fair

If you've ever been around children very long, you've probably heard them say, "That's not fair!" My own kids said it *zillions* of times, sometimes daily during those trying teenage years. But if we're honest, it's not only children who want things to be fair. It's human nature for all of us to long for fairness . . . and that can make the diagnosis of cancer especially difficult.

You may feel it's unfair for you or your loved one to have cancer because you're too young, or you've taken such good care of your body, or you've hardly been sick a day in your life, or you've already had to face cancer with another relative, or you have enough other problems.

I really believed—and still do—that my colon cancer diagnosis was *very* unfair. My good diet, exercise, young age, and healthy living should have prevented it, but they didn't. Every doctor I met shook his head and said I had done everything right *not* to get cancer.

Cancer is very unfair. Even if you "did" something to get it or didn't do something *not* to get it, it's still unfair. Maybe you are a smoker diagnosed with lung cancer. Cancer is still unfair, because only about 20 percent of smokers develop lung cancer. Maybe you quit smoking twenty or thirty years ago and you still got cancer. Hardly fair.

Perhaps you didn't get regular mammograms, Pap smears, or PSAs, and now you have cancer. Guess what? It's still not fair, because lots of people don't get those screening tests and don't get cancer. Besides, some people get them faithfully and the cancer isn't even detected! That seems even more unfair.

I know so many people who have had to deal with a terribly unfair diagnosis of cancer:

Like Peggy and Nick, who married after both their spouses died, only to have Peggy diagnosed with multiple myeloma a month after their wedding.

And Michelle and Jamie, in their twenties, who six months after they said "I do" found Michelle had Hodgkin's disease and later learned a bone marrow transplant would leave her unable to bear children.

And Doris, who just got her mantle cell lymphoma in remission, only to be diagnosed with another rare cancer, leiomyosarcoma.

And Lynn, a never-smoked health nut, diagnosed with lung cancer at the age of forty-eight.

And Ron, whose mother and brother both died from cancer while he was fighting his own battle with colon cancer.

I don't know if I ever said it out loud after my diagnosis, but I definitely thought it many times: *This is not fair.* And another question I never voiced but really wanted answered: *If God really loved me so much, why did He allow an unfair thing like cancer to strike my life?*

Then I learned a life-changing lesson from author
Philip Yancey:

☀ *Don't confuse life with God.*

In Yancey's book *Disappointment with God*, he
writes about a man named Douglas whom he interviewed because he thought Douglas might feel great
disappointment with God. Life, as Yancey describes it,
had been very unfair to Douglas. While his wife was
battling metastatic breast cancer, Douglas was involved
in a car accident with a drunk driver and suffered a terrible head injury that left him permanently disabled,
often in pain, and unable to work full-time.

But when Yancey asked this victim of unfairness to
describe his disappointment with God, Douglas said he
didn't feel any and instead told Yancey the following:

> I have learned to see beyond the physical
> reality in this world to the spiritual reality.
> We tend to think, "Life should be fair
> because God is fair." But God is not life.
> And if I confuse God with the physical
> reality of life—by expecting constant good
> health, for example—then I set myself up for
> crashing disappointment. . . . If we develop

a relationship with God *apart* from our life circumstances, then we may be able to hang on when the physical reality breaks down. We can learn to trust God despite all the unfairness of life.[8]

Go ahead and say it.

☀ *It's not fair that I have cancer.*

☀ *It's not fair that my loved one has cancer.*

☀ *It's not fair that this has happened to us right now.*

☀ *Say it, but don't be confused that life should be fair because God is.*

☀ *Life is not fair, but God is not life.*

Dear Lord, I'm so disappointed that this cancer has touched our family. It feels so unfair. Please help me to accept that life has been unfair to us but still to believe that You will be faithful to us. Please help me to develop a relationship with You apart from my circumstances and to learn to trust You despite the unfairness of life. I pray this in Jesus' name. Amen.

DAY 12
David vs. Goliath

God doesn't give you more than you can handle.

Does that ring a bell? I hear it a lot, especially from cancer patients or their family members who are feeling overwhelmed. They usually say something like this: "Now, I know God doesn't give us more than we can handle, but . . ."

Many people are under the misconception there is a Bible verse that states this fact.

There isn't.

The closest thing I can find is 1 Corinthians 10:13, which says:

> *No temptation has overtaken you except what is common to mankind. And God is faithful; he will not let you be tempted beyond what you can bear. But when you are tempted, he will also provide a way out so that you can endure it.* (NIV)

I do believe that there is *never* a time we are tempted to sin when we simply have no choice but to give in. God always provides a way of escape so we can withstand temptation. The Bible also tells us that temptations do not ever come from God.

I also believe, however, that sometimes trials come into our lives that *are* more than we can bear on our own, and cancer often is one of them. I consider myself a strong person, but cancer and the prospect that my possibility of dying was greater than my possibility of surviving was more than I could face. Worrying about whether my daughters would have to grow up without a mother was way more than I could bear. And fearing that my husband would bury another wife was absolutely more than I could endure.

"This is more than I can handle," I remember telling God, trying not to sound too whiny.

"I know," He answered. "But it's not too much for Me."

That was one of the most freeing things I learned through my cancer journey. It was all right that I sometimes had more than I could handle. That's when I would see Philippians 4:13 come true in my life:

I can do all things through Christ who strengthens me. (NKJV)

I didn't have to reach down inside myself and muster up some super strength. God supernaturally supplied it to me as I trusted in Him.

What a relief!

☀ *Even if my own resources were exhausted, God's would never be.*

☀ *My strength might be sapped, but He could still move mountains.*

☀ *Everything could be changing around me, but He was always my Rock.*

During those first dark days after cancer, I often thought of the shepherd boy David as he went into battle against the giant Goliath. Do you know what his battle cry was? He wasn't like the Little Engine That Could, chugging along and repeating, "I think I can, I think I can."

No, I believe he was thinking, *I know I can't, I know I can't.* He was the youngest and smallest boy in his family. Goliath was more than nine feet tall. But David's battle cry was, "I know God can, I know God can." If you read 1 Samuel 17:47 (NIV), you'll see his exact words: "The battle is the LORD's." That phrase appears many times throughout the Old Testament, and it was what I said to myself as I awoke on most post-diagnosis mornings.

"I feel like a little shepherd with a slingshot facing a giant named Cancer, and it is more than I can handle," I told the Lord. "But I am so glad it is not more than You can handle. The battle belongs to You, Lord. Fight for me and through me. Do what I cannot do on my own."

And He did.

I love how the apostle Paul describes a time in his life when he was faced with more than he could handle:

> We think you ought to know, dear brothers
> and sisters, about the trouble we went through
> in the province of Asia. We were crushed and
> overwhelmed beyond our ability to endure, and
> we thought we would never live through it. In
> fact, we expected to die. But as a result, we stopped
> relying on ourselves and learned to rely only on
> God, who raises the dead.
>   2 CORINTHIANS 1:8-9

Sometimes you may get more than you can handle in your own strength. That's okay. Whatever has happened to you has not taken God by surprise or caught Him off guard. He's prepared for the battle and will equip you with whatever you need not to become a victim of this giant called Cancer but instead to become a victor over it! Stop relying on yourself and learn to rely on God.

Thank You, Lord, that even when life gives me more than I can handle, it's never too much for You. When I am weary or worried or overwhelmed, remind me that You have what I require to face each moment and that You will supply all my needs as I trust in You. In the strong name of Jesus. Amen.

DAY 13
Taken by Surprise

I don't think most people are prepared to get a cancer diagnosis. Instead we hope against hope that things will not turn out as we fear and the whole nightmare will go away. Right up until I saw the look on my gastroenterologist's face after my colonoscopy, I had hoped—and believed—there was nothing wrong with me. So much for the power of positive thinking!

My friend Sandy says the first emotion she felt after hearing her diagnosis of advanced ovarian cancer was disbelief.

"I was sure they had the wrong diagnosis and they must have gotten someone else's report," the retired schoolteacher recalls. "I kept thinking the doctor would call in a few days and clear everything up."

I don't know if your or your loved one's cancer diagnosis has taken you by surprise, but I guarantee it has not taken God by surprise.

☀ *He is all-knowing.*

☀ *He is all-seeing.*

☀ *He is all-powerful.*

☀ *He is in control of everything.*

☀ *He knows what you need and when you need it.*

You may feel unprepared, but God is prepared, and He is preparing things for you—good things—things that you can't even imagine.

> *No eye has seen, no ear has heard,*
>   *and no mind has imagined*
> *what God has prepared*
>   *for those who love him.*
>   1 CORINTHIANS 2:9

And I believe He literally goes before all of His followers into each new day to provide what we'll need

for that day. Hear His promise through Moses' words
in Deuteronomy 31:8 (as expressed in three different
Bible versions):

*The LORD himself goes before you and will be
with you; he will never leave you nor forsake you.
Do not be afraid; do not be discouraged.*[9]

*GOD is striding ahead of you. He's right there with
you. He won't let you down; he won't leave you.
Don't be intimidated. Don't worry.*[10]

*Do not be afraid or discouraged, for the LORD will
personally go ahead of you. He will be with you;
he will neither fail you nor abandon you."*[11]

Authors Henry and Richard Blackaby explain God's
promise this way:

God never sends you into a situation alone.
He always goes before His children, as He
did with the children of Israel when He led
them with a cloud by day and a pillar of fire
by night. . . . He always precedes you in any
situation you encounter. God is never caught
by surprise by your experience; He has already

been there. He is prepared to meet every need because He has gone before you and knows exactly what you will need for your pilgrimage.[12]

And the really good news is that He doesn't just go on ahead of us; He stays with us, too, ensuring we are never alone. The Blackabys add:

Not only does God go *before* you, but He also stands *beside* you and *behind* you, to provide protection and comfort. . . . If you are going through a difficult or confusing time, know that your Lord has gone before you and He is present with you. He is fully aware of what you are facing, and He is actively responding to your need.[13]

God knows exactly what you need to be prepared for today.

"My faith got me through each day," Sandy recalls three years after her diagnosis. "I am truly a wimp when it comes to things like needles, blood work, and surgery, but the Lord gave me daily what was needed. I learned that He does not give us strength or grace the day before it is needed, but at the exact second it is needed."

It's okay if you feel disbelief or shock or are unprepared for whatever's next. Perhaps you would like to pray with the psalmist today from Psalm 25:5:

Lead me by Your truth and teach me, for You are the God who saves me. All day long I put my hope in You. Amen.

DAY 14
Inside a Cancer Storm

I've read that the eagle, like many other animals, can sense a storm before it arrives. So the eagle flies to a high spot and waits for the inevitable winds. When the storm hits, the eagle sets its wings so that the wind will pick it up and lift it above the storm. While the storm rages below, the eagle is soaring above it. The eagle does not escape the storm but uses the storm to lift itself higher. It rises on the winds that bring the storm.

God has allowed a storm of cancer in your life, and He *will* give you His strength to rise above it until He ultimately calms it.

Those who trust in the LORD will find new strength.
They will soar high on wings like eagles.
ISAIAH 40:31

If you feel that soaring above the storm is hard work, uncomfortable, and sometimes downright scary, you are right. That's why I use the analogy of a storm: we might not mind one from a distance, but it's not exactly pleasurable when we're smack-dab in the middle of a big one.

In fact, flying in a storm is extremely dangerous. My cousin Jim knows this from his half-dozen years of soaring into hurricanes and typhoons as part of a US Air Force weather reconnaissance team. It was his team's job to gather weather data so forecasters could better predict a storm's strength.

As they worked, it was critical that team members trusted the "artificial horizon"—a line on the plane's instrument panel that always corresponds to the earth's horizon, no matter in which direction the plane is flying.

"When you're in the clouds and in storms and you can't see the horizon—the earth, the ground, good old terra firma—you have to rely on the artificial horizon," Jim explains. "You have to trust that it *is* representing the horizon. You have to trust that it represents something you can't see."

Because of the extreme variability of the weather, there are two government ratings for pilots: one group is cleared to fly only when there's good visibility—following Visual Flight Rules (VFR)—and the other is cleared to fly even in poor visibility because they can keep a plane controlled solely on the data from their instruments—by Instrument Flight Rules (IFR). If you recall, after John Kennedy Jr.'s fatal plane crash, the National Transportation Safety Board said the young pilot—who was rated to fly only with VFR—had become disoriented in the night sky and lost control of the plane.[14] Experienced pilots are taught to rely on their instrument panel—no matter how they feel—because they can become so disoriented in clouds or during a storm they may think they are flying up when they actually are heading down.

In the early days of aviation when aircraft had few navigational aids, a successful flight was accomplished mainly by the pilot's judgment and instincts; that is, "flying by the seat of your pants."

"All you could do was fly by your sensations," Jim explains. "If you were coming out of your seat, you must be upside down. If you were pressed down into your seat, you must be flying higher.

"The problem is that our perceptions are not always accurate. You can *feel* like you're flying normally and are perfectly fine, but it's just that the airplane is *falling* at just the right speed that feels normal. You have to look at your instruments and believe them."

Flying by the seat of your pants through your cancer storm isn't a good idea either. Feelings can be overpowering and paralyzing. You may become so disoriented you don't know whether you're headed up or down.

That's why you need to decide every day to trust the magnetic poles of the earth—in other words, to recognize that God's Word is the compass on your instrument panel in the storms of life. It is truth, which, just like the pilot's artificial horizon line, always will point you in the right direction.

> *When the storms of life come, the wicked are*
> *   whirled away,*
> *   but the godly have a lasting foundation.*
>   PROVERBS 10:25

> *Put your hope in the LORD.*
> *   Travel steadily along his path.*
>   PSALM 37:34

I love author Max Lucado's perspective: "Faith is trusting what the eye can't see. . . . Eyes see storms. Faith sees Noah's rainbow."[15]

Dear Lord, it's hard not to focus on the storm around me. Please help me to trust that the promises in Your Word are more reliable than my feelings. Give me the strength to rise above this storm and even the faith to see a rainbow. In Jesus' name. Amen.

DAY 15
Hurry Up and Wait

When I ask cancer survivors what was hardest about the first weeks after diagnosis, many say the waiting was the worst.

"First it was waiting for the mammogram," recalls my friend Kristie, who, just shy of her fortieth birthday, discovered a breast lump. "Then it was waiting for the results of the mammogram. Then it was waiting for the appointment with the surgeon. Then it was waiting for the results of the biopsy. Then waiting for several other doctors' appointments for second opinions and consultations.

"All the while every doctor we saw said, 'This needs to be taken care of as soon as possible,'" recalls Kristie. "The medical world's perception of 'soon' and ours was miles apart!"

My friend Bill recently shared with our support group that his wife, Joan, was really discouraged immediately after her mastectomy as she waited to regain her physical strength and return to her normally energetic routine.

"I told her she just needed to be patient," recalls Bill, "but she told me, 'I've already been patient for two days—I'm tired of being patient!'"

I am convinced that those of us who are planners (like Kristie, Joan, and me), who like to be prepared and who relish being in charge, make the worst "waiters" on the face of the earth. Waiting prevents us from planning, impedes us from being fully prepared, and thwarts our attempts to be in control of the present as well as the future.

I've learned I need to be thankful for waiting. I know, I know . . . I'm thinking the same thing as I type these words: *You've got to be kidding! Why should we ever be thankful for waiting?*

Because waiting reminds us that we aren't God, and that's an invaluable lesson for all of us. We, of course, would never declare, "I am God." But every time we get impatient, annoyed, and frustrated with waiting, we demonstrate our need to be in charge. When we wait for others, it puts us at their mercy. They are controlling our schedule, our pace of life, and our agenda. Things are out of our hands.

Let's be honest: most of us do not want to be at the mercy of someone or something else. But the Bible tells us that we are at God's mercy for every breath we take.

> *In him we live and move and exist.*
>   ACTS 17:28

And every time we have to wait on God to answer our prayers, it reminds us that we are at His mercy.

☀ *Waiting goes against our very nature but draws us closer to the Lord better than just about anything else.*

I have some advice for you. It's the same advice I tell myself when things are taking too long. When you're waiting, don't give up—give in . . . to God. Go ahead and put yourself at His mercy. That's where you already are anyway. You might as well admit it, because when you do, then you can start to experience the transforming power that waiting can have on your character.

Don't get confused. It's not that the waiting itself changes us—otherwise we all would be pretty wonderful people. After all, everybody has to wait sometime! But it's how we *respond* to the waiting that can be transforming.

I love how author-pastor Rick Warren explains in *The Purpose Driven Life* that godly characteristics—things like love, joy, peace, patience, kindness, goodness, faithfulness, gentleness, and self-control—are developed in our lives when we are put in situations in which we are tempted to respond in exactly the *opposite* way. "Patience is developed in circumstances in which we're forced to wait and are tempted to be angry or have a short fuse," Warren writes.[16]

I put this principle into practice one day recently while I braked for yet another red light on my hurried lunch-hour errand trip. I looked straight at the light, smiled, and said out loud to myself, "I am not waiting for a traffic signal. I am being conformed into the image of Jesus!"

The declaration made me laugh out loud. But I'll tell you, it was a wonderfully freeing moment. I didn't squirm waiting for the light to change. I wasn't frustrated that I wasn't making good time. I just sat there and enjoyed the presence of God, which supernaturally settled over me.

Try it yourself.

☀ *I am not waiting for test results; I am learning to depend more on God.*

☀ *I am not waiting for a doctor to call me back; I am learning to be patient as God is patient with me.*

☀ *I am not waiting in cancer's shadow; I am becoming more like Jesus.*

Feel better about waiting? Just in case you need a little more encouragement about the positive benefits of waiting, I've compiled a list of my favorite verses on the subject on page 209. I hope you'll memorize a couple of them to encourage yourself the next time something or someone is taking too long! There is no faster way to wait, but there is a better way.

I'd love to pray for patience for *both* of us today:

Heavenly Father, it's so hard to wait. Please use these forced delays to transform us to be more like You. In Jesus' name I pray. Amen.

DAY 16
Defying the Verdict

"Don't defy the diagnosis; just defy the verdict."[17]

That sentiment from author Norman Cousins has become a sort of rallying cry for my cancer support group members who are facing especially difficult circumstances. These are the folks who realize that shock and disbelief—although understandable reactions to a diagnosis—can't really do anything to *change* the situation. So they decide to take the bull by the horns and refuse to give in to any statistics on a piece of paper or doomsday predictions from a doctor's lips.

So just in case you or your loved one has been given some not-so-great cure odds or perhaps even *no* odds for a cure, I encourage you to quit fighting against the diagnosis and instead to fight the verdict. Even if you or your loved one has great survival odds, I think you'll be blessed by today's story of a patient defying the odds.

My German-born friend Jutta (pronounced *you*-tuh) was diagnosed with Stage 3 pancreatic cancer at the age of thirty-eight. It's an understatement to say that cancer of the pancreas is not a "good" kind of cancer, and it's especially scary when your children are only six and ten. But that was the situation in which Jutta found herself in July 2003.

She felt fine and hadn't even considered that the jaundice she was experiencing might mean she was seriously ill. The day after exploratory surgery discovered a malignant pancreatic tumor had already spread to the lymph nodes, Jutta's surgeon came into her hospital room and told her, "You'd better get your act together. You have cancer, and you've only got two years."

Jutta was shocked not only at the diagnosis, but at the less-than-compassionate way the news was delivered.

"It took me at least a month to get over that," she says. Eventually she decided the doctor's prediction was only that—a prediction—and she would not live believing it *had* to come true. Good thing—as I write this, it is eight years later, and Jutta has never had a recurrence and remains cancer-free.

As she reflects on her cancer journey, she says, "You don't stop living just because you hear the word *cancer*. That's the worst thing you can do. Even if my cancer had been Stage 4, I would have still set goals and gone for them. I believe that somebody who sets goals lives longer."

Jutta says she still has a goal of being "an encouragement to other people." And you can bet I tell every new pancreatic patient I know about her!

When I was diagnosed, I was told I had about a 40-, maybe 50-percent chance of surviving. It seemed to me as if someone were going to flip a coin: heads I live, tails I die. It drove me crazy thinking about it.

And then a basic truth hit me: God wasn't playing roulette with cancer.

☀ *He didn't have His fingers crossed.*

☀ *He wasn't going to wish me luck.*

☀ *He wasn't taking bets on my future.*

☀ *He didn't need good odds to heal me.*

You need to know and believe that cancer is not an automatic death sentence. Doctors do their best at predicting cure rates and odds of survival, but these predictions are just educated guesses. When my friend Linda's kidney cancer spread to her lungs, her doctor told her she had six months to live. She looked him in the eye and responded, "I don't see any expiration date stamped on me." That was five years ago, and she was at our support group last month!

I'm very glad that my oncologist does not regularly dole out predictions about how long patients have to live. He feels those predictions become self-fulfilling prophecies in many patients' minds. I know zillions of people who have lived longer—some many times longer—than doctors or medical science predicted.

Predictions are just that. They do not have the last word. Please remember today that your and your loved one's times are in God's hands and He doesn't need "good odds" to heal.

In the words of the late pastor/author Charles L. Allen, "When you say a situation or a person is hopeless, you are slamming the door in the face of God."[18]

Lord, please keep us all from slamming the door in Your face; from refusing to believe that You are the God of the unexpected, the improbable, and even the impossible. Thank You that You have power over everything—over every errant cell in our bodies, over every discouraging word on our lips, and over every hopeless thought in our minds. We open the door to You and the healing touch You want to bring to our lives. In Jesus' name. Amen.

DAY 17
There's Always Hope

I love Jutta's advice to set goals because I think it helps those of us facing cancer to be able to celebrate many triumphs along this journey. If your *only* goal is for you or your loved one to be cured, it might take quite a while to reach that goal because, frankly, physicians aren't eager to use that C word with cancer patients. I bet it was at least ten years after my diagnosis before a doctor finally described me as a *cured* patient.

So go ahead and set your long-term goal to be cured, but set some other, shorter-term goals along the way.

My friend Jim has done this as well as anyone I know. When he was diagnosed with a glioblastoma multiforme (translation: the deadliest brain cancer) in July 2006 at the age of fifty-nine, no one gave him much hope. The golf-ball-size tumor affected his left side, and he had to learn to walk and talk again after surgery. When the tumor recurred just four months later, no one gave him any hope at all.

But Jim, a Vietnam veteran with two Purple Hearts, was desperate to live as he was caring for his wife, Jean, who also had advanced cancer. When I saw him in our office, he told me the doctors at the Hershey Medical Center thought he might have only three months to live. I suggested he "try to defy the verdict" and set some goals for himself.

"What would you like to be alive to see?" I asked him, thinking he'd choose something happening in the next few months.

"I want to see my son Travis graduate from college," he quickly replied.

"Okay," I said. "What year is he now?"

"A freshman."

Uh-oh. I suggested that perhaps Jim should pick a closer goal so we could celebrate sooner (while thinking there was *no way* this patient was going to be alive in four years!). So we decided on his daughter, Abby's, wedding in six months. Realistically, there was no reason to expect Jim to live even that short time, but it was a good goal, and I told the radiation tech next door that Jim wanted to walk his daughter down the aisle in the spring.

"I don't think there's much chance of that after looking at his tumor," the tech replied honestly.

Jim got radiation and oral chemo, but the mass persisted. Every time I saw him over the next few months, we talked about the impending wedding and prayed for Jim to be there—even if his hair wouldn't. On May 12, 2007, the prayer was answered, and Jim brought me the wedding photos to prove it!

Then a couple of months later, he went on a clinical trial drug because there was no other treatment available and set a new goal of holding his son Ryan's first child due in October. Both Jim and Jean got to hold that little grandson, and an MRI in January showed Jim's tumor had decreased slightly. But the joy was short-lived as Jean passed away in August 2008. Our clinical staff bemoaned that Jean's four children undoubtedly would be burying both parents in a short span of time. But Jim continued to defy the verdict. He set another goal of seeing Abby's first child born (she wasn't even pregnant yet!).

Bimonthly MRIs continued to show Jim's tumor shrinking, and in May 2009, he joyfully announced that Abby's little daughter, Lillian Jean, had arrived. Then an unexpected joy came: the next month's MRI showed the tumor was gone! That fall Travis entered his senior year of college, and Jim set his sights on seeing that graduation.

In May 2010, despite all odds, Jim was there to watch his youngest son awarded his college diploma.

But then he faced a new problem.

"What's my goal going to be now?" Jim asked me afterward.

"I guess you need to see Travis get married and have some kids," I volunteered.

"Sounds good," he replied.

And that's where things stand as I write this. Jim remains in an unexplained complete remission—five years since his diagnosis. I'm thinking we may need to set a goal of Jim seeing his *great*-grandchildren!

When Jim was first diagnosed with a brain tumor, he was angry, disappointed, and frustrated, especially over the fact that he was told he had such a short time to live. What gave him hope, he said, was hearing about others who had survived brain tumors or had lived much longer than doctors expected.

"I thought if they can do it, why can't I?" he recalls. "I was most thankful for people encouraging me and telling me there was still hope. And without my faith in God, I don't think I would be here now."

I can't promise God will answer your prayers exactly as He did for Jim, but I can promise that He hears the longings of your heart and wants to show you His great love today. Whatever your goals are, "let love be your highest goal" (1 Corinthians 14:1) and believe that God has good things in store for those who love Him.

Thank You, God, that You are able to do even more than we can ask or imagine. We lift our hopes and dreams to You, believing You will do what is truly best. In Jesus' name. Amen.

DAY 18
Families Facing Cancer

When I was diagnosed with cancer, our daughters were only eight, ten, and twelve, so my husband and I desperately wanted to protect them from cancer's assault on me. At first we thought it would be best *not* to explain my diagnosis. So we decided we would tell them I was going to have surgery but wouldn't use the word *cancer*.

That bright idea lasted about twenty-four hours until I realized that somebody in our church or small community was going to use the word *cancer* and my girls would hear it. So we sat them down again and using the dreaded "big C" word, we tried to give them an idea of what to expect. We were careful not to give them too much information that would scare them, but also not to make promises we couldn't keep.

We didn't promise that "Mommy is going to be fine" because we knew there was no such guarantee. We did, however, assure our girls that "the doctors would do everything possible to make Mommy better" and "Mommy would do everything she could to get better." We, of course, did not share with them that the cancer was locally advanced and that I had about a 40-percent chance of cure.

And with that brief but emotionally painful conversation, we had our children place their hands in ours, and together we placed all of our hands in the Lord's as we began to walk my journey with cancer together.

It was the best decision we could have made because time and again our daughters were able to see what it means to trust God in hard times. They learned better how to pray and wait on God, and as the months and years have gone by, they have seen how God can use even awful things for His glory.

If you still have children at home—or even grandchildren nearby—you have a perfect opportunity to show them your faith in action. It's easy to talk about things like the power of prayer and trusting God, but a diagnosis of cancer in the family gives us a chance to see if our walk matches our talk.

In those first, really dark days after my diagnosis, I remember feeling as if I wanted to go to bed, pull the covers up over my head, and have somebody call me to come out when it was all over. But I also remember my head talking some courage into my faint heart.

You've always told your children:

☀ **God can be trusted.**

Now they can see if you really do trust Him.

☀ **God is faithful.**

Now they can see if you will be too.

☀ **Knowing Jesus makes all the difference.**

Now they can see if it really does.

We were a family, and that "for better or for worse" pledge my husband and I made applied to our children, too. Together we would face cancer with the courage that God would pour into each of our hearts supernaturally, no matter our age or bravery status.

It is a much more powerful lesson for children to walk *with* you firsthand as you deal with cancer in your life or a loved one's life rather than hear about the journey later, after the fact.

They need to see that you are afraid sometimes and learn how you find courage.

They need to hear that you have worries and discover where to find hope.

They need to know that you don't have all the answers and observe how to talk to the One who does.

They need to believe that when God and cancer meet, God always is more powerful.

Whether He takes the cancer out of the person or the person out of the cancer, He gives every believer the victory.

Cancer was probably the best real-life lesson to prove to my kids that God can and will meet our deepest needs—that He can give us courage to face things we never thought we could. I'm so glad we decided to allow our family to walk that difficult journey together.

Father, I wish I could shield the children in our family from even thinking about cancer. But instead, help us to face this diagnosis together and to trust that You love them even more than I do. Please pour Your peace into their young hearts. Amen.

DAY 19
Unexplainable Peace

Everybody reacts differently to the diagnosis of cancer. Your reaction and mine probably had many things in common, but no doubt there were differences as well. You might have feared cancer for years because other relatives already had been diagnosed. Maybe you checked for lumps and watched for telltale signs, knowing for certain your turn was next. Or you might have thought, like I did, that you had taken such good care of yourself you would *never* have to face such a diagnosis.

I'm guessing that neither of our reactions was completely peaceful. I've met literally thousands of newly diagnosed cancer patients, and I've yet to hear one say, "As soon as I heard it was cancer, I felt total peace." (Go ahead and write me if you said that!)

But even though peace is not a natural response to a life-threatening illness, it can be a supernatural one.

Over the years my dear friend Prudence let me bring hundreds of cancer survivors to her country tearoom for free or really inexpensive tea luncheons (with the world's best scones and clotted cream). And then endometrial cancer struck her.

"That upset me," she says. "I didn't want to have anything inside me that wasn't supposed to be there."

But shortly after her surgery, despite the fact that no one was guaranteeing a cure, Prudence says she amazingly "was at peace with it."

"Christ gave me a wonderful release from worrying and obsessing about it" is her explanation of the unexplainable.

In 1998, when forty-five-year-old Chrystine was diagnosed with late-stage ovarian cancer, she was shocked and afraid she would die because she'd never heard of any survivors in her situation. But as she puts it, "God showed up right away."

As she was heading into surgery, a female anesthesiologist came over to Chrystine's gurney and started prepping her.

"She told me she had ovarian cancer four years before, and I felt such hope that she had survived," Chrystine recalls.

What's really incredible is that a few minutes later a male anesthesiologist came over to her gurney and told the other doctor that Chrystine was *his* patient, and he took over her care.

"I went into surgery feeling totally at peace because God sent me hope in the 'accidental' meeting of an anesthesiologist who had survived," Chrystine says.

It is one thing to read the apostle Paul's description of "the peace of God, which transcends all understanding." It's quite another thing to see it on the face of cancer patients and their caregivers.

☀ *It is a peace that makes no sense.*

☀ *It is a peace that cannot be explained.*

☀ *It is a peace that goes beyond our human understanding.*

☀ *It is a peace that only God can give.*

☀ *It is a peace I hope you'll feel today.*

I'd like to share with you the rest of the passage from Philippians 4, where Paul writes about this peace, because I believe it shows us clearly how to get it:

> *Do not be anxious about anything, but in*
> *every situation, by prayer and petition, with*

thanksgiving, present your requests to God.
And the peace of God, which transcends all
understanding, will guard your hearts and your
minds in Christ Jesus.
   PHILIPPIANS 4:6-7, NIV

We get peace from God when we take our worries to Him in prayer, all the while thanking Him for all our blessings. He replaces our worries with His peace, and it is enough to fill our hearts and our minds.

Would you allow me the precious privilege of praying for you to feel God's peace that passes understanding today?

Lord, I have no idea what is troubling my friend today, but You do. By the power of Your Spirit, please let Your peace come and settle down on her/his life as she/he trusts in You. In the name of the Prince of Peace. Amen.

DAY 20
Amazing Cancer Patients

I knew her as "the Horse Lady" long before I knew her name was Nicola.

And if I were writing a brochure about amazing

things cancer patients have done while undergoing treatment, the Horse Lady would be my cover photo.

She got her nickname from Marc, who initially had trouble remembering her name but had no trouble bragging about her exploits to me even before I worked in his office. His favorite story was about how she loaded up one of her prized thoroughbred horses in her horse trailer, hitched it to her pickup, and drove all the way from Pennsylvania to Oklahoma. After delivering the horse to its new owner, she continued to drive herself to Mexico for a vacation.

"Drove the truck herself with her oxygen tank right beside her on the front seat," Marc said with a satisfied smile. "She's amazing!"

I've met a lot of amazing cancer patients.

I know a man who earned his green belt for karate while being treated for lung cancer. I know a woman who went to dance class wearing a belt pump that released a continuous infusion of chemotherapy into her while she danced. I know another man who won a racquetball tournament a couple of days after his treatment for widespread colon cancer.

My friend Leanna started running 5K races *after* her diagnosis of Stage 4 melanoma. She's not super fast, but at age sixty-eight, she's usually quick enough to win her age category!

"I thought I'd give it a try to see if it would help me get better," says Leanna, a grandmother of eleven who still works part-time babysitting neighborhood children and is in complete remission from the cancer. She's even convinced her husband, Larry, seventy, to compete in an upcoming race with her.

"He was going to enter in the 'Clydesdale' category for men who weigh over 200 pounds," she says, "but I told him he might have a better chance of winning the seventy-plus category in case there's a young guy who weighs over 200 and is really fast!"

Our office even has our own version of Lance Armstrong with a patient named Eric, who was diagnosed with testicular cancer in 1987 at the age of thirty-one. Like Lance, Eric had Stage 4 disease, which had spread to his liver, lung, and groin by 1988. Now, twenty-four years after his diagnosis, Eric remains cancer-free and is enjoying life with his wife and three grown children.

You've probably seen the little yellow "Live Strong" wristbands from the Lance Armstrong Foundation. They're a neat way to remind cancer patients and their caregivers that a little ol' thing like cancer couldn't stop Lance from winning seven consecutive Tour de France cycling races. (No matter what controversy surrounds him, there's no doubt he's an incredible athlete and an amazing cancer survivor.)

I was sad, though, when I read in Armstrong's first book, *It's Not about the Bike*, that he doesn't believe in God, but rather only in himself and in his ability to be "essentially a good person."[19] He gives God absolutely zero credit for his recovery from cancer or his athletic accomplishments.

Personally, I think God supplies supernatural strength to us many times when we don't even realize it and that the reason our bodies have an amazing ability to heal is because He created us that way.

So while I agree with Lance that cancer patients and their caregivers need to live strong, I like even better the affirmation adopted by my friends Barry and Barbara when she was facing pancreatic cancer:

☀ *"By His Strength."*

Barb's younger brother Tommy even bought silver bracelets for all the family members with the letters "BHS" engraved on the front. The bracelets were partly a Christian response to the "Live Strong" wristbands. But mostly they were a reminder that this family intended to live strong by God's strength—even if they always didn't have the fortitude within themselves.

The initials BHS always reminded Barb's family of their heavenly Father and of their earthly family: Barbara Hall Streeter and Barry Howard Streeter.

Perhaps you feel 100 percent confident in your own abilities to face and conquer cancer, but there must be a little room for concern or you probably wouldn't be reading this book.

Isn't it good to know that you don't always have to have it completely together, you don't always have to just tough it out, and you don't always have to conjure up your own courage? Instead, at those times when you feel inadequate—or even hopeless—you can live "By His Strength."

I love how *The Message* Bible paraphrase describes Abraham's response when God told him He was going to make him the "father of many nations" even though Abraham and his wife, Sarah, were way past child-bearing ages:

> *When everything was hopeless, Abraham believed anyway, deciding to live not on the basis of what he saw he couldn't do but on what God said he would do.*
>
> ROMANS 4:17

☀ *Don't be discouraged by whatever you—or doctors or medicine—can't do, but live on the basis of what God says He will do.*

> *Joyful are those who have the God of Israel as their helper,*
> *whose hope is in the LORD their God.*
> PSALM 146:5

Lord, I do want to live strong, and I want to do it by Your strength. I'm so grateful that You have what I need to get through each day. In Jesus' name I pray. Amen.

DAY 21
Just in Time

My friend Polly has been on a personal journey with cancer for more than eight years, although her family's trek with this dreaded disease stretches back decades. Her mother, several maternal aunts, and her sister all had breast cancer, and the nagging thought of it was always there in Polly's mind too.

So when she got the same diagnosis at age forty-eight, she was anxious and upset, but not really surprised. The shock came four years later, in 2007, when the cancer returned and spread to her lungs and bones (and no, I haven't forgotten my happy-ending promise—keep reading!).

"I thought I was a goner," she recalls. "I kept thinking, *I hope I have another birthday.*"

Polly had the lung tumors removed and started more chemo. We talked and prayed often, and Polly kept drawing closer to God as she sat on her front porch each day watching hummingbirds, reading the Bible, and talking with her heavenly Father in prayer.

Four months later, the PET scan showed significant improvement, and two months after that, all signs of the cancer were gone. Two and a half years later, she remains in an unexplained, *complete* remission despite stopping all treatments several months ago.

"It's a blessing beyond my wildest dreams," she says. "It's been a wonderful journey of a whole new closeness with the Lord. He just knows what I need right now—this minute, this hour.

"I have learned to seize each day," she adds. "Every day I get up and say, 'You can have a good day or a bad day,' and I always choose good."

I believe Polly has been experiencing what it's like to walk with God as He goes before you and lights your way during the dark times. Don't expect that He will light up your *whole* journey—He might reveal just the next few steps. And don't imagine that His provision will arrive way ahead of time so you can stockpile it until you're ready to use it.

If you know the Old Testament story of the Israelites wandering in the desert for forty years, you'll remember God sent just enough manna—a grain-like food—for each day (see Exodus 16). If they tried to gather extra to save for the next day, the leftovers turned moldy—except for the day before the Sabbath, when they were permitted to collect a double portion that still would be fresh the next day. It has been my experience that God continues to provide for His people, like my friend Polly, just what we need in the nick of time—not way ahead, as most of us would like!

My favorite illustration of God's perfect timing is a story shared by Corrie ten Boom, the Dutch Christian concentration camp survivor whose family helped hide Jews from the Nazis during World War II. The conversation she relates took place when she was a little girl and her father tried to calm her fears that she would be unprepared when she had to die someday:

> Father sat down on the edge of the narrow bed. "Corrie," he began gently, "when you and I go to Amsterdam—when do I give you your ticket?"

I sniffed a few times, considering this.

"Why, just before we get on the train."

"Exactly. And our wise Father in heaven knows when we're going to need things, too. Don't run out ahead of Him, Corrie. When the time comes that some of us will have to die, you will look in your heart and find the strength you need—just in time."[20]

☀ *"Don't run out ahead of Him."*

What marvelous advice. God needs to go *before* us into each day. We don't yet have what we need to face all of our tomorrows, because we are not yet there. But every day as we come to our heavenly Father in prayer, He promises to guide us and provide for us in that minute, that hour, that day.

I pray you'll have faith in Him—the kind of faith Moses showed the Israelites when he knew he could not lead them into the Promised Land where they would face powerful enemies. I'd like to pray for you today Moses' words of encouragement from Deuteronomy 31:6, spoken to a group of worried people who feared the unknown:

*Do not be afraid and do not panic before them. For
the LORD your God will personally go ahead of you. He will
neither fail you nor abandon you. Amen.*

DAY 22
Already a Survivor

So when do you know that you or your loved one is
a cancer survivor? When the scan comes back clear?
When the tumor marker is normal? When the treatment is finished? When there's no evidence of any
cancer?

I was diagnosed June 26, 1990, with Stage 3 colon
cancer. I still am cancer-free and count myself as a very
blessed survivor. But even if the cancer had returned,
I would still count myself as a survivor because I agree
with the National Coalition for Cancer Survivorship
when it labels cancer patients as survivors "from the
moment of diagnosis and for the balance of life."

I didn't always think that way.

I used to think that if you lived five years cancer-free
after a diagnosis, you were a cured cancer survivor.

I remember going in for my five-year oncology
checkup in the summer of 1995 (before I started

working in Marc's office) and gleefully announcing to Marc that I wouldn't be seeing him professionally anymore. (I'm not quite sure how I got that notion, but I hear many others say the same kind of thing. We've probably made that association because statisticians often give data on five-year survival rates for different types of cancer.)

"Where did you get that idea?" Marc responded.

"It's five years; I'm cured!" I told him, surprised that he didn't realize it was such a momentous day.

"Well, the chance the cancer will return has diminished greatly, but you still need to be checked for the rest of your life," Marc soberly explained.

Talk about bursting someone's bubble!

I had waited five years to be proclaimed a survivor, and there was going to be no such official announcement.

Thankfully, a short time after that day, I read the above-mentioned survivorship definition from the National Coalition for Cancer Survivorship and proclaimed myself a survivor.

So I hope you're not waiting for some mythical five-year mark to earn the label of cancer survivor. Anyone who has survived even one minute since diagnosis already is a survivor! Believe it!

I love watching and listening to those survivors in my support group who have medically incurable cancer but still find much happiness. Because of their circumstances, others might say these folks have the right to be fairly fearful. But these "incurable" survivors have come to realize—as have those of us who are cured—that we don't need the right circumstances to be happy, but we do need to *believe* the right things about our circumstances to be happy.

It's important what you believe about yourself and your loved ones. When I finished treatment for my cancer, the odds the cancer would come back were *greater* than the odds it wouldn't. That doesn't sound like a situation that would make a person very happy. But what I believed about my circumstances did give me joy.

I believed the truth that I was already a cancer survivor.

> *As he thinks within himself, so he is.*
>   PROVERBS 23:7, NASB

And I believed the truth that nothing, including cancer and its treatment, can diminish God's great love for me.

I am convinced that nothing can ever separate us
from God's love. Neither death nor life, neither
angels nor demons, neither our fears for today nor
our worries about tomorrow—not even the powers
of hell can separate us from God's love.
  ROMANS 8:38

I also believed the truth that God didn't need good
odds to heal me, that there are people everywhere surviving despite their odds.

Nothing is impossible with God.
  LUKE 1:37

You and your loved ones have survived a cancer
diagnosis. God obviously has plans for your life or you
wouldn't still be here. Ask Him to shine His light on
your path, and then don't be afraid to follow where
He leads.

Will you pray from Psalm 119:105-107 with me?

Your word is a lamp for my feet and a light for my path.
I've promised it once, and I'll promise again: I will obey your
wonderful laws. I have suffered much, O LORD; restore my life
again, just as you promised. Amen.

DAY 23
Laughter Therapy

I've read that "laughter is like changing a baby's diaper—it doesn't permanently solve any problems, but it does make things more acceptable for a while."

And while there's nothing funny about cancer, I have discovered that every time a person facing cancer laughs, it reminds us that we are still alive, and that is a very good thing. I am a firm believer that we all need to keep—or get—a sense of humor as we walk our cancer journeys.

So if you're tired of worrying and would like to laugh a little today, I'd like to introduce you to my friend Dorothy, one of those really great people with the ability to make the most out of life's embarrassing moments even though she lived in cancer's shadow for many years. I know her funny story won't permanently solve any problems in your life, but I think it will feel really good at least for a little while to "have your diaper changed"!

Dorothy, a widow nearing eighty and facing recurrent cancer, wasn't the type of patient who was easily discouraged. In fact, she told me in March 2003 that her surgeon had predicted that she had only three months to live when he had operated on her twenty-eight months earlier!

"I feel I still have work to do. Besides, I don't have the sense to give in," she added with a big smile.

And she did not give in. Instead, she fought her disease with the help of new chemo, supportive family, and the healing medicine of laughter. Invariably when she would come into our office, Dorothy would have a hilarious story to share—usually about her wig.

I remember the funniest story she ever told was March 21, 2001—I know the exact date because afterward I ran to my office and wrote it down word for word as best I could remember it. I knew I would never want to forget this one.

Dorothy said that after her last treatment, she felt a little hungry and decided to drive to a nearby restaurant called Claire's, famous around town for its broasted chicken and fresh peach sundaes. She parked near the door on the side of the restaurant, which had large picture windows for customers to gaze out on the parking lot.

As she stepped out of the car, she felt the elastic in the waistband of her slacks snap. Not wanting her now-too-loose slacks to slide down, she quickly grabbed the waistband with her right hand. As she did, a huge gust of wind came up and—you guessed it—blew her wig right off her bald head.

Of course, Dorothy lunged for the wig but it got away. She did, however, manage to set off the car alarm on the keys she still held in her tightly clenched hand, which also was holding up her slacks.

Picture this: the car's lights flashing, the horn honking, the slacks still slipping, and the curly, platinum blonde wig still blowing away as Dorothy, a completely bald, five-foot-nine-inches-tall octogenarian, runs across the parking lot.

"I kept frantically trying to punch buttons on the keys to turn off the alarm, but I didn't want to drop my drawers," she said. "My wig just looked like a little tumbleweed as it rolled across the parking lot."

Finally it came to rest against a truck tire, and Dorothy started talking to the wig as she ran closer: "You might as well let me catch you now because if you blow under the truck, I'm crawling under there to get you, and you won't get away!"

Apparently the wig believed her and stayed put until she could grab it.

She plopped the little tumbleweed back on her head and finally found the right button to turn off her car alarm.

"What did you do then?" I asked when I could get a breath after all the laughter.

"I got in the car, put it in reverse, and drove across town to McDonald's," she said. "I may never go to Claire's again!"

Every time I drive by Claire's, I smile as I picture Dorothy chasing her wig that day. I imagine there are probably some customers who witnessed the event and still relish retelling the story!

Laughter is good for the body. Science is just figuring that out, but the Bible told us long ago:

A cheerful heart is good medicine,
but a crushed spirit dries up the bones.
PROVERBS 17:22, NIV

Tomorrow I'll share some specific ways to strengthen your funny bone, but for today just remember you only need *one* reason to be happy:

This is the day the LORD has made.
We will rejoice and be glad in it.
PSALM 118:24

Father God, help us to rejoice today simply because we're alive. Let us find joy in life no matter what our circumstances may bring. In Jesus' name. Amen.

DAY 24
Strengthening Your Funny Bone

About a month before my diagnosis I was a reporter for a local paper and writing a story about the new cancer support group at the local hospital. I interviewed Marc for the story and visited his office. When I walked by the chemo room, I glanced in at all the patients in recliners hooked up to IVs. It was an incredibly scary picture to me. But what was even scarier was that the patients were *laughing*. I remember thinking that they must not know they had cancer because how could people with cancer ever laugh? I went home that day and told my husband, "If I ever had cancer, I definitely would not be sitting there laughing."

Four weeks later when I was diagnosed with colon cancer, I definitely was not laughing. When I went for my first chemo treatment in August 1990, I was so frightened I knew I would *never* laugh while hooked up to an IV getting toxic chemicals.

But that was before I met Marc's head chemo nurse, Ruth, who had been with him since he opened his office in 1989. I can't recall what silly thing she uttered, but before I knew what had happened, she had me laughing too.

There was still nothing funny about having cancer or getting chemo or not knowing if I would see my daughters grow up, but every time I laughed it felt so good and reminded me that I was still alive.

So I decided I needed to keep my sense of humor and started to look for funny things *in spite of* my serious predicament.

One of the first things my family found to joke about was the new chemo pill I took—levamisole. It was a newly approved oral medicine, and I was the first patient at Marc's office to take it. I soon learned that in reality it was a worming medicine designed to kill intestinal parasites in sheep and dogs.

Whenever I took a pill, I started barking and chasing my squealing daughters around the house. My husband mentioned to our friends that I had been dewormed and he was thinking of getting me a rabies shot too. The pills were very expensive, and my husband often suggested we call the vet to see if we could get them cheaper there. (A regular comedian, huh?)

My support groups have a reputation for a lot of laughing, and every time we laugh together, it reminds us that we are still alive . . . and that always is worth cele-brating. If you don't have a funny oncology nurse or a laughing support group nearby (or a comedian hus-band!), here are a few suggestions to "strengthen your funny bone" from former MLB pitcher and cancer survivor Dave Dravecky's ministry newsletter:

- *Start your own comedy collection of jokes and car-toons.* (Do an Internet search for "clean jokes," and you'll find some good laughs. Post them at your desk or on your fridge so you can remind yourself to laugh.)

- *Get your groceries and get a chuckle.* Read some of the tabloid headlines while standing in the check-out line. (I just read about aliens with anorexia and manure as a miracle cure for arthritis!)

- *Hang out at the greeting card racks.* Enjoy perusing funny cards (wash your hands first, and don't eat an ice cream cone while you do this!). You can even buy a comical card to brighten someone's day. (One day at work I received a card with an odd-looking old man on the front, which said, "I bet I can still float your boat . . . even if I don't have both oars in the water!" It was from my wonderful husband to cheer me up.)

- *Become a humorous-people groupie.* Hang out with funny people, like my dear friend "Grandma" Doris, a seventy-nine-year-old, three-time colorectal cancer survivor, who often livens up our meeting introductions by wearing goofy glasses or showing off her silly souvenirs. (Either you're a funny friend or you need one!)

- *Make the most of embarrassing moments.* (Did I tell you about the time a pair of my underwear dropped out of one of the pant legs of my jeans onto the floor of a Christian bookstore while I was shopping there? . . . Never mind.)

In his book *The Purpose Driven Life*, Rick Warren writes that our first purpose in life is to please God. Or as Warren puts it, "The smile of God is the goal of your life."[21]

Cancer can and often does take things away from us and from our families, but it needn't take away our goal in life—to please God, to make Him smile.

No matter what you've gone through or what still lies ahead—whether you have no cancer, a little cancer, or a lot of cancer—will you choose joy? Will you choose to please God and bring a smile to His face? It is your choice. You can choose to keep (or get) a sense of humor even in cancer's shadow.

I have a prayer of blessing for you from Numbers 6:24-26 as you try to find joy today:

May the LORD bless you and protect you. May the LORD smile on you and be gracious to you. May the LORD show you His favor and give you His peace. Amen.

DAY 25
Circle the Wagons

I remember so well the first cancer support group meeting I attended at our community hospital. As I mentioned yesterday, I was a reporter for a local newspaper, and in addition to interviewing Marc for my story about the new support group, I also had interviewed the group's facilitator, Mary. Two months later when I showed up at a meeting, Mary naturally assumed I was visiting the group as a follow-up to my published article.

"How sweet that you would come to our meeting," she said with a big smile.

"Actually, I was diagnosed with colon cancer last month," I told her as her jaw dropped.

It was an incredible irony.

I had to talk myself into attending that meeting because I wasn't sure I really wanted to be with a bunch of people with cancer. As introductions were made around the table, I happened to be the most newly diagnosed and the last to introduce myself.

I burst into tears before I could even get out my name.

I felt silly for falling apart like that, but I had been trying to hold it together in front of everyone else for so long that it seemed good to let down my feelings with others who had "been there, done that."

In the more than twenty years I've run my own cancer support group, I don't think I've ever had a new person who didn't cry or at least get teary at the first meeting—and that includes all the men, too!

My friend Chris, diagnosed with an astrocytoma brain tumor in 1999 and still cancer-free, says what initially gave her hope was a cancer support group actually called H.O.P.E. (Hope for Oncology Patients & Encouragement). Soon she began attending my Cancer Prayer Support Group as well and found it "very comforting to get together with others who were going through a similar experience."

"We can all talk about things we can relate to and others might not understand so well," she adds. "And what I still find very helpful is that we actually laugh together and have a great time. Yes, there are times we cry together, but we've actually been asked to keep down the [laughter] noise when there are other meetings going on in rooms near us!"

After my friend Ken was diagnosed with tongue cancer in 2002, he believed for a while that he wouldn't need things like support groups.

"I assumed that because of my [spiritual] faith I wouldn't need other forms of support such as groups, family counseling, and massage therapy, but I was dead wrong," Ken explains.

Many years later and still cancer-free, Ken urges newly diagnosed patients not to try to go it alone.

"Circle the wagons—family, friends, coworkers, and anyone else who can and will be an available asset in your battle," he says. "You can never have too many assets!"

I'm always inviting cancer patients and their caregivers to my support group meetings, and I hear a lot of reasons why they don't attend. Often people tell me, "I'm not really so depressed that I need to come."

To which I reply, "I need people there who *aren't* depressed to support those who are!"

I believe there are two reasons for people to attend support groups—either to be encouraged or to be an encourager. And I'm pretty sure you could fit into one of those categories! I encourage you to find a faith-based cancer support group (I'm compiling a state-by-state list on my website, www.lynneib.com) or to think about starting one of your own in your area (free information to do just that also is available at my website).

The apostle Paul describes how God once sent someone to encourage him when he was down and out.

> *When we arrived in Macedonia, there was no rest for us. We faced conflict from every direction, with battles on the outside and fear on the inside. But God, who encourages those who are discouraged, encouraged us by the arrival of Titus. His presence was a joy.*
> 2 CORINTHIANS 7:5-7

☀ *Never forget that we serve a God who "encourages those who are discouraged."*

When Paul "faced conflict from every direction," God sent his friend Titus at just the right time to fill him with joy. God knows exactly what you need in order to deal with today's discouragement. Ask Him to bring a Titus (or two) into your life to encourage you. (He might even direct you to a support group with a bunch of Tituses!) And maybe someday you'll be just the encourager someone else needs to meet.

Dear God, please lead me to people who understand what I'm going through and who will encourage me on this journey. Help me not to depend on my own strength, but to lean on others who have walked this walk and can give me hope. In the name of Jesus. Amen.

DAY 26
Positively Not Positive

You can beat this. Think positive. You can do it. Stay positive.

I know people mean well when they say those things to cancer survivors, but I must admit they often rub me the wrong way.

Many caring people uttered those kinds of "encouraging" phrases to me after my cancer diagnosis, but I often had the feeling that they did more for the person saying them than they did for me.

In fact, rather than being comforting and encouraging, those phrases often created more distress in me.

I'm feeling worried the cancer may return, but I have to think positive so the cancer doesn't come back.

I'm feeling down thinking about all I've endured, but I have to think positive so I get healthier.

And the real kicker: *If I don't get cured, it must somehow be my fault because I didn't think positive enough!*

Don't get me wrong; I am by nature an optimistic person, but I am also positively positive that being positive *all* the time is not necessary for those living in cancer's shadow, and in fact I wouldn't even recommend it for most of us!

In fact, trying to live life by being "up" all the time can create a new problem: "the tyranny of positive thinking."

That's the phrase used by Dr. Jimmie Holland, chairman of the Department of Psychiatry and Behavioral Sciences at Memorial Sloan-Kettering Cancer Center. In her excellent book *The Human Side of Cancer: Living with Hope, Coping with Uncertainty*, she explains the phrase:

> All this hype claiming that if you don't
> have a positive attitude and that if you

get depressed you are making your tumor
grow faster invalidates people's natural and
understandable reactions to a threat to their
lives. That's what I mean by the tyranny of
positive thinking.[22]

The truth is, Dr. Holland says, "stress, depression,
and grief do not increase the likelihood that cancer
will develop or that it will come back if you've been
treated before."[23]

I can tell you for sure that if *not* staying positive
made cancer recur, I would have been dead many times
over.

Now if by some slim chance you are really the kind
of person who likes to think positive *all* the time, copes
with life by *always* thinking positive, and finds it *impossible* to think any other way, I certainly am not going
to tell you to *stop* thinking positive. But please, don't
expect that everyone else needs to be just like you.

I believe we were created to feel many emotions and
that life is best lived when we acknowledge those emotions and express them in a healthy manner. Moreover,
I believe tears are really a gift and that everybody—
even a positively positive person—benefits from a good
cry now and then.

If you ever tasted a tear trickling down your face,

then you know they are salty. But tears are much more than salty water. They're actually a complex combination of proteins, enzymes, lipids, metabolites, and electrolytes.

We all have three different kinds of tears: "normal" tears that continuously keep our eyes lubricated, irritant tears that wash away foreign substances, and emotional tears that we cry for reasons like sadness and pain. Scientists who study tears can look at these tiny drops of water and tell the difference between the first two types and the third kind because emotional tears have much more protein and less oil.

Some tear researchers theorize that emotional tears carry hormones from the brain, which release calming endorphins and flush toxins out of the bloodstream. This helps our body return to a reduced-stress state.

I'm glad my dear friend Norma was willing to cry with me throughout my chemo ordeal. Norma, now cancer-free in her nineties, has survived three different cancers. Her second diagnosis was just a few months before mine, and she called me every month to chat.

"Wanna have a pity party?" she'd ask.

I'd say sure, and for the next half hour we'd trade poor-me complaints about the side effects of our treatments. Pretty soon we'd had enough moaning and started laughing at ourselves for all the complaining we were doing. (The moral of the story: pity parties are great occasionally; just keep them short, and only invite friends who still like to laugh!)

People like Norma and me who don't repress our tears may have better health, according to many "crying" researchers who think emotional tears may remove toxins from our bodies. Some even theorize that women, on average, live longer than men because they, on average, cry twice as much!

Many of us need to tell ourselves the truth: that weeping is not a sign of weakness or shame, that tears are indeed a gift to express our deepest feelings. The shortest verse in the Bible is John 11:35: "Jesus wept." He was standing at the grave of his friend Lazarus, and He could have uttered some positive platitudes, but instead, Jesus cried. If the very Son of God can shed tears, I think we can too.

Lord, I'm thankful that one day in Heaven You will wipe away every tear from our eyes, and until then, I'm positively happy that we don't have to stay positive all the time! I pray in the name of Jesus, who wasn't afraid to weep. Amen.

DAY 27
Feeding Your Mind

So tell me the truth: when you read the obituaries, do you scan down to the bottom to see if memorial contributions are to be made to the American Cancer Society?

I know I did after my diagnosis. Every night I'd look in the paper to see if someone I had treatment with had died or how many people listed that day had died from cancer. It was a depressing ritual, but one I found hard to break. I guess it was part of those early days when I let cancer consume my thoughts.

It also seemed to me as if the word *cancer* came up daily in conversations or in the celebrity news headlines. If all that cancer was out there before, I never had noticed it. I guess it's like what happens when you get a new car and all of a sudden you notice lots of people with the same make and color vehicle.

And thank goodness I had cancer "in the olden days," as I like to call them, when I didn't have Internet access in my home or at my fingertips on a mobile device. I'm pretty sure that vast amount of web information would have made me feel even more overwhelmed. (I just Googled the term *colon cancer*, and 18.6 *million* sites came up!) Often when a newly diagnosed patient comes into my office for the first time, the patient's spouse will practically beg me to tell the patient to "stop reading everything on the Internet."

Don't misunderstand, I'm thrilled at all the information—and encouragement—that is available on the web, but a good question to ask yourself after your online time is, *Do I feel* better *or* worse *after what I've just read?* If information makes you feel better equipped to fight the cancer battle, then search away. But if information makes you feel overwhelmed or depressed or fearful, please don't keep putting such stuff into your head. (Much of it isn't accurate anyway!)

Instead I would encourage you to fill your mind with the truth that the God who created this universe by simply speaking words is a lot more powerful than any misguided cells within our bodies and is a lot more trustworthy than any statistics in a medical journal.

☀ *Stop feeding your mind with a voice of fear and instead allow a strengthening fear to fill your being.*

I'm talking about the fear of the Lord.

It's not a "fall down and shake because you're afraid of getting zapped" kind of fear, but a *Wow!* kind of fear. It's the kind where you are just in awe and amazement

and wonder and reverence about God because of what
He has done and still can do.

It's this "fear" that I and so many other cancer survivors have discovered *reduces* all the other fears.

I love how Psalm 112 describes us "fear-filled" kind
of people:

> *Happy are those who fear the LORD.*
> > *Yes, happy are those who delight in doing what he*
> > > *commands. . . .*
> *When darkness overtakes the godly, light will come*
> > *bursting in.*
> > *They are generous, compassionate, and*
> > > *righteous. . . .*
> *They do not fear bad news;*
> > *they confidently trust the LORD to care for them.*
> *They are confident and fearless*
> > *and can face their foes triumphantly.*
> PSALM 112:1, 4, 7-8

I remember watching my friend Anne triumphantly
face her cancer-foe back in 1994, when she was diagnosed with small cell lung cancer and Marc gave her
only a 10- to 20-percent chance of survival.

When I asked her what gave her hope throughout
her cancer journey, her God-fearing, God-trusting

reply was, "I thought, *If it's God's will, I can be in that 10 to 20 percent.*"

Near the end of her treatment, Anne also survived a harrowing bout with sepsis, which easily could have taken her life. Seventeen years later, she still is cancer-free and now the head chemo nurse in Marc's office.

The Old Testament prophet Isaiah explained how he, too, learned to have the right kind of fear after God warned him that his country was going to be invaded.

> *The LORD has said to me in the strongest terms:*
> *"Do not think like everyone else does. Do not be*
> *afraid that some plan conceived behind closed*
> *doors will be the end of you. Do not fear anything*
> *except the LORD Almighty. He alone is the Holy*
> *One. If you fear him, you need fear nothing else.*
> *He will keep you safe."*
> ISAIAH 8:11-14

I don't know about you, but that's one voice of fear I always want to hear.

Heavenly Father, please help me not to feed my mind with fearful things, but instead to confidently trust that You will care for me and my loved ones. Strengthen me not to fear bad news, and empower me with fearless confidence to triumphantly face this foe, cancer. Amen.

DAY 28
Hearing from Heaven

I hope you have someone who is praying with you during your cancer journey—not just *for* you, but right *with* you so you can hear your needs lifted to Heaven. Even though I have been privileged to pray with cancer patients and their caregivers for the past twenty-plus years, I never cease to be amazed when I see God answer. It's always especially exciting when patients tell me it's the first time they really heard from God.

Maureen was one of those patients.

It's easy to remember when I first met Maureen and her husband—it was the first anniversary of the September 11 terrorist attacks.

What a rotten day to have to start chemo, I thought as I talked with the couple in my office. Maureen was forced to reschedule this first treatment because the week before, she'd had to go to Nebraska, where her mother had taken ill while visiting relatives.

As I explained my job of offering emotional and spiritual support, I could see that Maureen was especially anxious regarding all that lay ahead. She said that she and her husband had gone to church early that morning to pray. I thought perhaps their visit was prompted by the day's special significance to our country, but she said they made the same visit most mornings before work.

However, Maureen admitted that she didn't feel she heard from God the way other people seemed to hear Him. Her husband concurred that the amazing things that happened to other people never seemed to happen to them.

I didn't have any answer to their dilemma but asked if I might pray for them before Maureen's first treatment began. They readily agreed, so we held hands and I prayed a prayer of blessing over them.

When I finished, Maureen had a shocked look on her face.

"I can't believe what you just prayed!" she said.

Oh dear, have I made some theological mistake? I wondered.

"Why? What did I say?" I asked her.

"You prayed that I would have 'strength, courage, and peace,'" she said. "Those are the three things I have been praying for, in that exact order, every day since I was diagnosed with cancer."

"So much for not hearing from God!" I responded with a smile. "I don't think there's any doubt now that He heard your prayers!"

I was pretty excited at God's amazingly fast answer

to this couple's desire to hear from Him, but He wasn't done with them yet that day.

Maureen went to get her IV hooked up, and I went into an exam room to talk with a patient named Dee. She told me she wanted to loan my first book to her next-door neighbor's daughter, who recently had been diagnosed with cancer. Dee added some details about how her neighbor had become ill while she was in Nebraska.

"Wait a minute," I said, stopping her story. "What's your neighbor's daughter's name?"

"Maureen," she replied.

I quickly dashed into the chemo room and asked Maureen for permission to introduce her to her mother's neighbor. Within moments, introductions were made between the two women who had heard much about each other but had never met. The veteran patient, Dee, hugged the novice patient, Maureen, and assured her she had been praying for her.

"I am so excited," Maureen kept saying. "Things like this never happen to me!"

And that's how Maureen learned for sure that God really did hear her prayers and that His amazing power wasn't just something that happened to other people.

I don't know if you hear from God every day or if you feel you've never really heard from Him, but I promise you that He wants you to draw close and hear His voice.

> *Oh, that we might know the LORD!*
>   *Let us press on to know him.*
> *He will respond to us as surely as the arrival of dawn*
>   *or the coming of rains in early spring.*
>   HOSEA 6:3

> *You faithfully answer our prayers with awesome deeds,*
>   *O God our savior.*
> *You are the hope of everyone on earth,*
>   *even those who sail on distant seas.*
>   PSALM 65:5

If you have someone who will pray with you, ask that person to help you hear from God. If you don't, please allow me that privilege right now:

Father God, my friend needs to hear Your voice today. Will You please somehow, in some way, speak to my friend in a manner that will show You do faithfully answer our prayers? In the name of Jesus. Amen.

DAY 29
Joining Club Paranoia

Have you noticed that when you joined the select group known as Cancer Survivors, you also got an unwanted membership in another group? I call it Club Paranoia.

This is the place where you feel nervous ignoring things that you never would have worried about before.

Where a dull headache might be a brain tumor.

Where a tiny old-age spot could be melanoma.

Where indigestion is possibly stomach cancer.

Where a backache surely is bone metastases.

Where lumps, bumps, aches, and pains seem much more pronounced right before your next checkup and much less right afterward!

One reason cancer survivors are so paranoid is because once our bodies have betrayed us, it's hard to trust them again. When I was diagnosed with cancer, I looked fine and felt fine. I certainly couldn't imagine I had a life-threatening illness. I thought that people with cancer would look sick or at least feel sick.

My theory in life used to be if you're not bleeding profusely or in terrible pain, you're okay. My parents, especially my father, who coached sports, always told me to "shake it off" if I got hurt as I was growing up. And that's what I continued to do as an adult.

So I have a little occasional blood in the stool. Probably an old hemorrhoid. I feel fine. Shake it off, I told myself. So my bowels are occasionally a little different. Probably something I ate. I look fine. Shake it off.

And that's what I did . . . for a year and a half. Both my family doctor (make that ex-doctor) and I ignored symptoms that I now know suggest cancer.

Perhaps you did the same. You ignored a warning sign or your doctor didn't seem too concerned about it, so you didn't bother with any tests. And now you want to make sure you never make that mistake again.

☀ Welcome to Club Paranoia.

A few years ago I had a little mole on my shin, which looked nothing like any picture of skin cancer I've seen (and believe me, I compared it to all of them). I showed it to two physicians and an oncology nurse— all of whom told me it did *not* look suspicious. Still, I made an appointment with a dermatologist to have it removed because it appeared suddenly and made me nervous. (It didn't help that my neighbor Sharon, much younger than I am, had a little mole on her leg, which also didn't look suspicious but turned out to be melanoma.)

Even if you were a hypochondriac before the cancer diagnosis, you're probably going to be a little more paranoid about the disease now. I have yet to meet a survivor who doesn't admit to at least some degree of irrational fear. I think cancer survivors and their loved ones *should* be suspicious and distrustful of cancer. It's a very sneaky disease and we are wise not to let down our guard when it comes to our health. That makes us smart, not paranoid.

It's the *irrational* fears we need to avoid. And we do that by being rational—by telling ourselves the truth about fears.

Most headaches are not brain tumors.

Most backaches are not cancer in our bones.

Most of the people diagnosed with cancer today can expect to still be alive five years from now.

Most cancer survivors are at least a little paranoid, and you're not crazy if you are too!

☀ **The truth is that while cancer cannot be trusted, God can.**

Let us hold tightly without wavering to the hope we affirm, for God can be trusted to keep his promise.
   HEBREWS 10:23

> *Trust in the LORD with all your heart; do not*
> *depend on your own understanding.*
>   PROVERBS 3:5

> *I prayed to the LORD, and he answered me,*
>   *freeing me from all my fears. . . .*
> *I cried out to the LORD in my suffering, and he*
>   *heard me.*
>   *He set me free from all my fears.*
>   PSALM 34:4, 6

You may not be able to completely cancel your membership in Club Paranoia, but you don't have to be a card-carrying member every day! (By the way, remember that little mole on my shin? The dermatologist removed it, and $184 later I found out it was not cancer. Did I mention that paranoia can be very expensive?)

Lord, I don't want to live a paranoid life, afraid that cancer is lurking around every corner. Please free me from this fear and help me trust in Your promises. I pray this in Jesus' name. Amen.

DAY 30
If God Is So Good . . .

When you believe in God, it can be hard to come to terms with the fact that He has allowed adversity to touch your life. Think about it.

If God knows everything, this diagnosis did not surprise Him.

If God sees everything, He saw the bad news coming.

If God has power over everything, He could have stopped it.

But He didn't.

He didn't stop you or your loved one from getting cancer.

Would you like to know why? Join the club!

My journalist friend Mike was awaiting the release of his first novel[24] when his colorectal cancer was diagnosed. At only thirty-five, with a wife and three young children, he wondered what God was doing (or not doing) in his life.

"Lord, in my head, I know You're in control, but my heart is wondering what's going on here," he said. "Are You sure You know what You're doing?"

My friend David Biebel talks about this dilemma

in his book *If God Is So Good, Why Do I Hurt So Bad?* He says there are two truths suffering people have to reconcile: sometimes life is agony, and our loving God is in control.[25]

In the beginning, it was hard for me to reconcile these truths. I honestly found that at first my faith made things *harder* rather than easier as I had to struggle with the fact that I had loved and faithfully served God for many years and yet He let something really bad happen to me when I knew He had the power to stop it. I've heard some people *without* faith respond to cancer very nonchalantly because they have kind of a "que será, será, whatever will be, will be" approach to life.

But for me, it's different. I don't believe that life is merely a series of random events that happen to us. I believe I have a heavenly Father who loves me, watches over me, and has good plans for my life. So why did a nice girl like me get a not-nice thing like cancer?

The reality is that God's Word never promises that He will stop all bad things from happening to us. On the contrary, it promises us that He is prepared for each battle and will equip us, too.

The Message paraphrases 2 Corinthians 4:8-9 this way:

*We've been surrounded and battered by troubles,
but we're not demoralized; we're not sure what
to do, but we know that God knows what to do;
we've been spiritually terrorized, but God hasn't
left our side; we've been thrown down, but we
haven't broken.*

☀ *God is in control.*

☀ *Errant cells aren't.*

☀ *Toxic medicine isn't.*

☀ *White-coated doctors aren't.*

☀ *Herbs and vitamins aren't.*

☀ *We aren't.*

Many of us would have to admit that we are "control freaks." We like to make plans, carry them out, and then smile at how well they went. We like to call the shots. We'd rather tell God what we think we need than have Him tell us. If we're truly honest, we may even admit that it's hard to pray for God's will because we know it may not be the same as ours.

Cancer can be a real wake-up call for us. We are forced to realize we are *not* in control of everything. But no matter how many (or how few) tomorrows doctors may have told you to expect, those tomorrows are safe because God is in control.

The sooner we learn this truth, the easier our fight against cancer will be. It's actually quite freeing once you get it right. You can relax knowing Someone else is in charge—Someone much more intelligent, powerful, and vigilant than we are or ever could hope to be.

Be encouraged that this health crisis has not taken God by surprise. He is in control and knows how to equip you for the fight. Will you pray from Psalm 31 with me?

O LORD, I have come to You for protection. . . . Be my rock of protection, a fortress where I will be safe. . . . I will be glad and rejoice in Your unfailing love, for You have seen my troubles, and You care about the anguish of my soul. . . . I am trusting You, O LORD, saying, "You are my God!" My future is in Your hands. Amen.

DAY 31
Eye of the Storm

The more I talk with my cousin Jim about his days of flying with an Air Force weather reconnaissance team, the more I believe that dealing with a cancer diagnosis is *a lot* like flying into a hurricane: both require an inordinate amount of trust.

Jim agrees with my observation and says it was difficult at first for him to trust he was going to be okay as his plane flew right into the eye of a storm.

"There's a lot of trust going on when you're going into harm's way," he explains. "You have to trust in the plane and the people who made it. You have to trust in the people who maintain the plane and that it won't fall apart. And you have to trust that the other crew members know what they're doing. And they all have to trust in you—that you will do the right thing too.

"But the more you do it, the more you know it's going to be okay," adds Jim, a retired USAF major, who has flown forty-four times into the eyes of hurricanes and typhoons.

Jim says the scariest part of the team's mission to gather weather data is the five or ten minutes just before the plane actually flies into the eye of the storm.

"You usually have to fly right through thunderstorms—which, of course, you normally would never do—and the turbulence is sometimes so severe you're really glad you're strapped into your seat," he explains.

But what happens next is so incredible it helps keep people like my cousin flying again and again into the eye of the storm.

"When you break through the eye wall, dramatically and suddenly the turbulence stops," Jim explains. "What was black and bleak is now sunny, quiet, beautiful, and really awe inspiring. There's blue sky above you, and you're like a little fish in the bottom of a bowl. You've found the exact, calm center."

Now I fully realize that, unlike my cousin Jim, you have not *chosen* to fly into a hurricane. I also realize I can't change the fact that your life has been touched by a cancer-storm. But I believe with all my heart that the Creator of the universe is able to lead you to the exact, calm center of that storm. I don't really understand how He does it any more than I understand how the middle of a hurricane can be beautifully quiet. But Jim has been there, so I believe him. The cancer survivors in this book—myself included—have many times found peace in the midst of our cancer-storms, and I hope you'll believe us, too.

> *Be still, and know that I am God!*
> PSALM 46:10

The word translated "still" is the Hebrew word *harpu*. I'm no Hebrew scholar, but I did some research and found it conveys the idea of being weak, letting go, surrendering, or releasing. It's the opposite of striving

with our fists up, ready to fight or at least defend ourselves. When we are *harpu*, our arms are at our sides,
relaxed.

And that's where we find the exact, calm center. It's
the place where we can relax in the tight grip of a sovereign God. We relax *not* because everything is okay,
but because we know the One who is in control . . . and
will one day in Heaven make everything okay.

Here's how some other Bible versions translate
Psalm 46:10:

Cease striving and know that I am God.[26]

Desist, and know that I [am] God.[27]

*Let be and be still, and know (recognize and
understand) that I am God.*[28]

*Our God says, "Calm down, and learn that
I am God!"*[29]

I hope one of these speaks to you today. I've included
them all because I'm such a word person and know that
words can resonate differently with each person. I'm
praying one of these renderings of this verse is just the
word you need to hear.

Personally, I really like the very literal translation to "cease striving." I tend to be an organized, driven person who really tries hard to get things worked out and doesn't do well being still and just relaxing in God's control!

May I pray for us both?

Heavenly Father, we don't do well being still. Help each of us to surrender our cancer-storms to You and trust that we can relax because You are in control. Give us the faith to let go and let You give us Your peace. In Your Son's name. Amen.

DAY 32
In Cancer's Shadow

There I was, staring right into the steely eyes of a hammerhead shark. Then another shark swam toward me. Over my shoulder, I could see a third heading my way.

I never flinched. I didn't even attempt to escape. In fact, I thoroughly enjoyed the whole experience.

Why? Not because I still had chemo-brain and didn't remember that sharks can be very dangerous. No, it was because I was completely protected from them.

The experience took place at the aquarium in Baltimore's Inner Harbor, and I was standing on dry ground watching the menacing-looking sharks swim past me in a huge, wraparound glass saltwater tank. They couldn't have touched me even if they had wanted to. So you see, it is possible to be surrounded by something life-threatening and yet feel very safe!

There's no arguing that cancer is a life-threatening disease. The shadow it casts on survivors and loved ones can at times seem very menacing.

In grade-school science, you may have learned that a shadow is caused by the absence of light when an opaque (not see-through) object has absorbed the light. When cancer casts a shadow in our lives, I believe it's blocking the light from reaching us. That's why I've shared all these true stories about cancer patients and their families—so you can believe that we truly can find the light despite cancer's shadow.

Another truth about shadows is that they fall *opposite* their light source. That's why your shadow is in front of you if the sun is behind you and vice versa. The way we're facing determines whether or not we can see the shadow easily.

I know this is a simple scientific fact, but it is a profound spiritual truth for cancer survivors and their loved ones. You have to keep facing the light in order not to see cancer's shadow so easily. You must keep turned in the right direction.

Do you remember in 1998 when the Galaxy IV communications satellite malfunctioned and rotated out of position, turning away from the earth? In an instant millions of pagers went silent, TV and radio stations couldn't transmit, and even some gas pumps couldn't accept credit cards. It all happened because just one satellite in the heavens turned the wrong way and couldn't communicate with Earth.

Perhaps when you first heard the diagnosis of cancer, you got out of position spiritually. You couldn't figure out how a loving God could allow cancer into your life. Maybe you even felt at times as if He didn't hear your prayers. I hope you will check to see which way you are facing now. The way to communicate with God is to be turned toward Him, pouring out our hearts to the One who hears, understands, and has the power to respond.

Once we're facing Him, talking to Him, and listening to Him, we can also *choose to live in a different shadow*. Now I know it sounds strange that you could find light by being *under* a shadow, but it's true.

The shadow I want you to move into—or stay in if you're already there—is a much, much bigger shadow than cancer's shadow. It's a safe, secure, protective shadow. There's no other shadow that can eclipse this one. And when we're in it, we're not in the dark; we're supernaturally in the light. You see, while the Bible describes God as light, it also refers to Him as a shadow, protecting us in His shade.

> *Those who live in the shelter of the Most High*
> *will find rest in the shadow of the Almighty.*
> PSALM 91:1

☀ **"The shadow of the Almighty."**

I love that word picture. Can you see yourself with a dark cancer cloud over your head, moving into the huge shadow of God Himself? Standing in the protection of His shadow, you can barely even see the little shadow-speck of cancer.

> *He has hidden me in the shadow of his hand.*
> ISAIAH 49:2

Have you ever put your arms around a child during a storm and drawn him close to you, protecting him from the rain and the noise? Have you ever seen a mother hen spread her wings and gather her little chicks to safety as danger approached? That's the picture that the Bible gives us of God's love and care for us.

How precious is your unfailing love, O God!
All humanity finds shelter
in the shadow of your wings.
    PSALM 36:7

May I pray for you?

Almighty God, please help my friend to live not in the
shadow of cancer, but in the protective shadow of Your
hand. And there let my friend feel Your unfailing love and
find rest. Amen.

DAY 33
Why Me?

Cancer helps you sort out who your real friends are. Often people you never realized cared for you step up and provide incredible support. And then there are those on whom you counted but now fail to come through for you.

My friend Kristie expected to get some words of healing and blessing when she went to talk to her priest shortly after a diagnosis of breast cancer sent her reeling just before her fortieth birthday.

She didn't get either.

"There was no comfort from him," Kristie recalls nearly twenty years later. "He told me, 'You deserved this. You've done something wrong, something bad, and this is God's way of showing you that.' He was adamant about it."

Obviously, Kristie went looking for encouragement in *other* places after that conversation!

Sadly, I have talked to many people over the years who thought—or at least wondered if—their cancer diagnosis was indeed a punishment from God. Usually there was something they did—or failed to do—and they thought the diagnosis might be God's response to that wrongdoing.

While I have no doubt that illness can get our attention and even spur folks on to change their sinful ways, I don't believe God is in the business of zapping people with cancer to get them to shape up. If doing something wrong or "bad" always led to cancer, everyone in the world would be needing to make an appointment with an oncologist!

Even in Jesus' time people were tempted to equate sickness with sin. Jesus' disciples once asked him: "Why was this man born blind? Was it because of his own sins or his parents' sins?"

Jesus' reply was clear: "It was not because of his sins

or his parents' sins. . . . This happened so the power of God could be seen in him" (John 9:2-3).

I never thought my cancer was a "punishment" for any of my sins, but I must confess I often wondered if I was "good enough" to be physically healed by God. Oh, I never doubted He *could* heal me, I just wasn't sure He would want to.

My doubts stemmed from an evil voice whispering in my ear: *Everyone prayed for Ralph's first wife, and she still died. You don't think you're better than she was, do you? If she wasn't good enough to be healed, you certainly aren't.*

Thankfully, my dear friend Sheila stopped by during this time and explained to me that my fight with cancer was a spiritual battle as well as a physical battle, and I needed to be reminded of Ephesians 6:16: "In every battle you will need faith as your shield to stop the fiery arrows aimed at you by Satan" (NLT1). Those "fiery arrows" often include depression, loneliness, fear, anxiety, and despair—all common emotions for people facing a life-threatening illness.

Sheila prayed with me and reminded me of the

truth I knew in my head but could not feel in my heart: God's love is not based on whether we're "good enough"—it is a gift, unconditional and with no strings attached.

Slowly but surely, I began to feel God's love again and to understand that my prayer for healing would not be answered as a reward for good behavior.

So I remind you today, neither you nor your loved one has cancer because you weren't good enough. And you *don't* need to do something special to earn or deserve healing from God. Don't try to bargain with Him by being an especially good person, hoping He will reach down and heal the cancer. There's nothing you can do to make God love you any more—or any less—than He already does. He proved that a long time ago:

> *This is real love—not that we loved God, but that he loved us and sent his Son as a sacrifice to take away our sins.*
> 1 JOHN 4:10

Author Max Lucado puts it this way:

> You wonder how long my love will last? Find your answer on a splintered cross, on a craggy

hill. That's me you see up there, your maker,
your God, nail-stabbed and bleeding. Covered
in spit and sin-soaked. That's your sin I'm
feeling. That's your death I'm dying. That's
your resurrection I'm living. That's how much
I love you.[30]

So if you're still searching for an answer to the why
question regarding your or your loved one's cancer, it's
not about you. Maybe, just maybe, it has happened so
that the power of God might be seen.

*Lord, thank You that You loved me first. And thank You
that I don't have to earn that love. I praise You for loving me
with an everlasting love and for proving it at the Cross. In
the name of our Savior Jesus. Amen.*

DAY 34
Attitude Adjustment

I'm the first to admit that I didn't have a very good attitude about being diagnosed with cancer. In my opinion I was too young, too healthy, too busy, and too
needed by my family to have this nasty interruption.

I'm usually a pretty positive person, but back then

the main thing I was pretty positive about was that I thought I was a goner. (Thank goodness the power of positive thinking failed me!)

It's often said that there are two kinds of people in life: optimists and pessimists. I want to remind you that optimism won't always change the inevitable. Take the case of the optimist who fell out of the twelfth-story window. As he went by the fifth story, he looked around, smiled, and said to himself, "So far, so good."

Pessimism isn't a very good idea either.

Did you hear about the farmer who lived next door to a pessimist? If the farmer said, "It's a beautiful day," the pessimist would reply, "We need rain." If the farmer was grateful for rain, the pessimist would reply, "It'll probably ruin the crops."

One day the farmer had had enough of his neighbor's pessimism and invited him over. The farmer threw a stick out to the middle of his pond. Immediately his dog went after it and walked on *top* of the water. He picked up the floating stick in his mouth, walked back across the top of the water, and laid the stick at the pessimist's feet.

The farmer looked at his neighbor and said, "Pretty amazing, huh?" to which the pessimist replied, "Can't swim, can he?"

You probably think I'm going to tell you to be an optimist. I am not.

I have found that the best attitude for a cancer patient is neither total optimism ("Without a doubt, I'm going to be cured") nor total pessimism ("Without a doubt, I'm going to die"), but positive realism ("Without a doubt, I have a life-threatening illness and I may or may not get better, so I will plan for both").

When we insist that we are going to be cured, we set ourselves up for a terrible defeat if that doesn't happen. On the other hand, if we insist our situation is hopeless, we already are defeated before we start. I believe it's best to be realistic and make plans to be financially, emotionally, and spiritually ready to depart this life. That's not giving up. It's coming to grips with our own mortality so we really can live life fully without fear of death.

I have seen scores of people who refuse to entertain the thought that they might not be cured of cancer because they want to remain totally optimistic. Those who weren't cured were devastated. I also know scores of people whose situations were medically hopeless, but they continued to live life fully, and some of them even went on to become cancer-free!

Please don't misunderstand me. I feel there is a difference between total optimism and a positive attitude.

Total optimism says, "I'm absolutely, positively going to be cured." A positive attitude says, "I hope and pray and truly expect that I'm going to be cured, but even if I'm not, I will not be defeated."

☀ *A totally optimistic attitude insists lemons will get sweeter. A positive, realistic attitude adds some sugar and makes lemonade.*

A positive attitude will help heal you—physically, emotionally, and spiritually—but it may or may not cure you. As a cancer support group facilitator and a cancer patient advocate, I've seen plenty of people with wonderful, positive attitudes who didn't get better, and I've seen people with crummy attitudes doing quite well. If we're honest, we all must admit that we have known people with great attitudes who did not get well from cancer or myriad other illnesses.

There were many days after my diagnosis that I shed tears and many days I held private pity parties for myself, but I did try to take control of my heart's attitude. So much else was out of my control: What chemo drugs I needed. How often I needed to take them. What their toxicity was. What my medical prognosis was.

I had no control over any of those, but I could control my attitude.

I love how author Chuck Swindoll describes the importance of attitude:

> Words can never adequately convey the
> incredible impact of our attitude toward
> life. The longer I live the more convinced
> I become that life is 10 percent what happens
> to us and 90 percent how we respond to it.
> I believe the single most significant decision
> I can make on a day-to-day basis is my choice
> of attitude.[31]

I can't guarantee that a good attitude will give you more *quantity* of life, but it definitely will give you—and those around you—more *quality* of life.

The heart of a cancer survivor—your heart—needs to find the right attitude.

Lord, please remind me today that what happens in me is more important than what happens to me. Send Your supernatural power to transform my attitude. In Jesus' name. Amen.

DAY 35
Worried about Worrying

Before I had cancer I really wasn't much of a worrier. When people would tell me they were worried about something, I would very *sensitively* tell them, "Well, just don't think about it."

After my diagnosis, I became a professional worrier. It's hard not to worry when people are always feeling you for lumps and checking you for recurrences.

At one point shortly after I finished my chemo, I found a lump on my neck. (This came soon after I talked with a friend who'd had thyroid cancer.) I kept pressing on this lump, and sure enough, it got sorer and sorer. When I went for my next recheck with Marc, I mentioned the sore lump. He felt it and politely told me, "Quit pressing on this lump or you will die. You're pressing on your carotid artery and you're cutting off the blood supply to your brain!"

I worried about other things, like my husband being widowed again and my daughters growing up without a mother. I worried that each holiday was my last and that I would never feel normal again. I knew it wasn't good to worry, so I worried because I worried so much.

But it's hard to stop worrying.

The more I tried *not* to think about cancer, the more I thought about it.

I remember the first day I didn't worry about cancer. It was a couple of months after my diagnosis, and I was a newspaper reporter engrossed in a story I was writing on my laptop. All of a sudden I looked at my watch with amazement—I had gone a whole two hours without thinking about cancer.

That was the beginning of my learning the secret to not worrying: something else has to occupy my mind. Philippians 4:8 says:

Fix your thoughts on what is true, and honorable, and right, and pure, and lovely, and admirable. Think about things that are excellent and worthy of praise.

When other thoughts came into my mind, worrisome thoughts, I asked myself if they fit these criteria: true, honorable, right, pure, lovely, admirable, excellent, or praiseworthy. If not, I pushed them out and replaced them with a thought that did. For me it was usually one of God's promises from His Word. When you want to empty your mind of worry, you have to have something encouraging to put in its place.

Another way to combat worry is not to look too far

down the road. Holocaust survivor Corrie ten Boom wrote, "Worry does not empty tomorrow of its sorrow; it empties today of its strength." That is so true.

When the phrase "what if" pops into your mind, you know peace is about to leave you. About 90 percent of the things I worried about never came true. Most of the what-ifs never happened.

In April 1997 I was faced with a possible what-if. An episode of irregular vaginal bleeding led to a sonogram, which showed a growth wrapped around my ovary.

"Probably just a benign cyst"—which I have a history of. "We'll watch it for three months," my gynecologist said, and I agreed. But a couple of days later, she called me back at work.

"I discussed your case with my colleagues, and they all feel this is an abnormal growth and it needs to come out," she said.

"What do you think it is?" I asked.

"Probably nothing," she said, "but it could be ovarian cancer or a recurrence of the colon cancer." I felt my stomach tightening. I tried to remain calm and nonchalant.

"We'll need to have a general surgeon on hand in case it is a colon recurrence and you need more surgery," she added. We went over pre-op details and I hung up.

All of the worries and fears I thought I had conquered after almost seven years were back.

In my job as a patient advocate, I encourage patients emotionally and spiritually, reminding them that God can be trusted no matter what the circumstances. Now I would find out again if I could trust Him in spite of *my* circumstances.

It took me about forty-eight hours, but I remember sitting in my bedroom and saying to God, "Okay, I don't like this one bit. I think it stinks. I don't want to die, and I don't want to go through more chemo. But God, You have proven Yourself so faithful in my life and have blessed me so much through my cancer experience, I would be nuts not to trust You now. So whatever is ahead, I know You are in control and I trust You."

Peace immediately flooded my mind. (P.S. The tumor was benign.)

The mind of a cancer survivor—your mind—needs to find peace.

My prayer for you today is that you would experience the peace of God as the apostle Paul writes in Philippians 4:6-7 (The Message):

Don't fret or worry. Instead of worrying, pray. Let petitions and praises shape your worries into prayers, letting God know your concerns. Before you know it, a sense of God's wholeness, everything coming together for good, will come and settle you down. It's wonderful what happens when Christ displaces worry at the center of your life. Amen.

(Still feeling a little anxious? Turn to page 211 for more hopeful verses on the subject.)

DAY 36
Surrounded by Hope

Not many seventy-seven-year-old women are upset about having cancer because they won't be able to tap-dance, but my friend Linda sure was.

The lively great-grandmother was diagnosed with primary peritoneal cancer (a rare female cancer usually treated similarly to ovarian cancer) in October 2010 and faced major abdominal surgery and chemotherapy. She knew those treatments were going to cramp her active lifestyle.

"I was a bit disappointed I was not going to be able to attend my once-a-year visit to my daughter's first-grade classroom and help her students make applesauce and tap-dance for them," explains Linda. She started tap dancing when she was about eight and in her mid-sixties still performed with a local group of senior ladies—ages fiftysomething to eightysomething—called "The Glitter Bugs."

But even worse than not being able to dance was Linda's worry that she wouldn't be well enough to take care of her ninety-two-year-old husband, who was in hospice care.

"My husband always thought of me as a 'spring chicken' who would be there to care for him, and when all this happened, he realized I might need some care too," Linda recalls.

So from the start of her cancer journey, Linda realized how much she was going to need her faith, her family, and her friends. Fortunately, she was surrounded by hope—literally.

That's because several years ago she started collecting items with the word *hope* on them. She has books, plaques, candleholders, Christmas decorations, flowerpots, and garden stones all proclaiming hope. In fact, everywhere she turns in her house or her yard, she sees hope! Four freestanding, silver letters—H-O-P-E—about five inches tall are her favorite decoration because she says she can easily move them to any area where she wants a visual reminder not to give up.

"I can't remember exactly when I started collecting, but I know there came a time when I realized our *hope* in God is what allows us to believe in something we do not see," Linda says.

And Linda doesn't just *collect* hope; she studies it too (and capitalizes it when she writes about it!).

"I had a ladies' Bible study on hope," she recalls. "Before the ladies came, I asked them to write down a list of things they hope for. We shared some of our hopes and kept others to ourselves. Inevitably somewhere on each list was the hope of Heaven."

At the end of the study, Linda gave each participant a handmade bookmark with her acrostic on HOPE:

Heaven
Offers
Peace
Eternal

"If we believe that, fear is diminished and even wiped out!" she says. "What peace we find in that hope!"

I agree completely with Linda that the promised hope of Heaven for all believers is what gives lasting peace. I love how *The Message* describes this hope in Hebrews 6:18:

*We who have run for our very lives to God have
every reason to grab the promised hope with
both hands and never let go. It's an unbreakable
spiritual lifeline, reaching past all appearances
right to the very presence of God where Jesus,
running on ahead of us, has taken up his
permanent post as high priest for us.*

That is the hope in which Linda continues to walk
on her journey with cancer. As I write this, it's only
been seven months since her diagnosis, but follow-up
tests continue to show her to be cancer-free. She knows
the odds are not in her favor, but thanks God "for my
remission time, however long it may be."

I think Zephaniah 3:17 is a beautiful description of
my *beautiful*, silver-haired friend Linda:

*With his love, he will calm all your fears.
He will rejoice over you with joyful songs.*

Perhaps you might want to embrace Linda's hobby
and start "collecting" hope—look for it and listen for
it each day. You'll probably be amazed at how often it
pops into your life. And I hope, like Linda, that you
have grabbed on to the promised hope of Heaven with
both hands and that you never let go.

Then you will be able to pray today as the apostle Peter did in Acts 2:25-26 (quoting King David):

The LORD is always with me. I will not be shaken, for he is right beside me. No wonder my heart is glad, and my tongue shouts his praises! My body rests in hope. Amen.

P.S. I'm happy to tell you that at our last support group meeting Linda reported she plans to tap-dance this fall and make applesauce with her daughter's new first-graders.

DAY 37
Money-Back Guarantees

"To what do you attribute your survival?"

That was the question posed to me this week by a newly diagnosed cancer patient. He's just a little younger than I am and undergoing chemo for "my" kind of cancer, so we have a special bond.

I thought about his question for a moment before I answered: "The grace of God."

I'm guessing he might have been a little disappointed with my reply as he's been researching all kinds of complementary treatments and nutritional advice for his cancer fight. I imagine he was hoping I had a vitamin regimen or a diet modification he could adopt.

I did tell him that throughout my treatment I drank green tea but always wondered if the honey I put in it was canceling out the tea's benefits. I told him about the supposedly cancer-fighting vitamins I took—at least one of which researchers now say may *cause* cancer rather than cure it. I told him how my husband and I grew all our own vegetables without any pesticides for years. I mentioned that I cut the sugar out of most things, left the skins on lots of things, and I added wheat germ to just about everything. ("Some crunchies on your cereal this morning, girls?")

I was a real health nut *before* I got cancer. In fact, I was pretty disappointed that all those doughnuts my husband ate and I passed up hadn't seemed to help me keep cancer at bay. I think subconsciously I even believed that my healthy eating and exercise routine would *guarantee* that I wouldn't be sick—after all, I hadn't had a cold for four years when I was diagnosed with cancer!

So when people ask me what I did to get cured, I refuse to give credit to anything I did or didn't do. I did what the doctors advised (well, most of it), but I felt so nauseated that I ate whatever tasted good rather than what had the best nutritional value. A short walk was all the exercise I could muster because I was too weak and had too many problems with an allergic reaction to one of my drugs.

I honestly don't know for sure why I'm still here. I feel uncomfortable suggesting that I did something *right* to survive cancer because that would mean that my dear friends who did not survive must have done something *wrong*.

That's why I say it was the grace of God.

After my diagnosis, I remember desperately wanting guarantees. I wanted to hear that the chemo regimen I was getting had a money-back guarantee, not a 20-percent chance of working on me. I wanted to know for certain that it was going to be all right to refuse the radiation some doctors had recommended for me. I wanted to be assured that if I went through all this difficult treatment, the cancer would not come back.

I didn't get any of these guarantees. And I can tell you that I've stopped looking for guarantees here on this earth.

You may be trusting in doctors or medical science or alternative therapies for a cure, but despite what you read, they *don't* have guarantees.

About the only earthly guarantee I can give you is that all of us *will* experience difficulties, including the breakdown of our physical bodies. But I promise you—more important, Jesus the Messiah promises you—we can face these difficulties with unshakable assurance, remaining deeply at peace. Why? Because Jesus has overcome the world by overcoming the power of death in our lives. Jesus already has beaten cancer and every other illness that strikes us on this earth.

And His kind of peace isn't just the absence of striving; it's the presence of something much more. The Bible says it this way:

> *I've told you all this so that trusting me, you will be unshakable and assured, deeply at peace. In this godless world you will continue to experience difficulties. But take heart! I've conquered the world.*
> JOHN 16:33 (THE MESSAGE)

Now that's a guarantee I can live with!

Let's pray today with King David from Psalm 20:7 (NIV):

> *Some trust in chariots and some in horses, but we trust in the name of the LORD our God. Amen.*

DAY 38
Trying to Be Thankful

When I was getting chemotherapy, my friends at church were excited that I was being treated by a physician who had strong spiritual faith and often asked me, "How did this little town manage to get a Messianic Jewish oncologist who is so well trained and respected in his field?" I used to reply jokingly that God sent him here just for me.

Now I know there was much more truth to that statement than I could have fathomed at the time.

A diagnosis of cancer, or any life-threatening illness, normally brings with it many emotions. Thankfulness is not usually on the list. When I found out my cells had gone awry and allowed cancer to grow inside me, gratefulness was the *last* thing I felt.

But I kept thinking about the admonition in the Bible to "give thanks in all circumstances" (1 Thessalonians 5:18, NIV). I knew enough to understand that did *not* mean I had to be some sort of masochist and praise God for every awful thing that happened to me. Instead, I believed it meant I could have a thankful heart no matter how depressing my circumstances were.

So a few weeks after my diagnosis, I began to look for something for which to be thankful. It was another one of those conversations between my head and my heart.

Let's see . . . I have cancer at the age of thirty-six after taking good care of myself physically. No, can't think of anything worthy of thanks there.

My three little girls may have to grow up without a mother. Nope, that doesn't work either.

I'm going to have to take toxic chemotherapy when I don't even like to take an aspirin. Not much there to feel grateful about.

Finally, it came to me.

Dr. Hirsh! I have a Messianic Jewish oncologist—who knows, maybe the world's only Messianic Jewish oncologist—practicing medicine just seven miles from my home. I humbly bowed my head and heart, and for the first time since hearing the dreaded news, "You have cancer," I thanked God in the midst of my circumstance.

"Father, You know I don't feel any happiness about my situation, but I want to thank You for leading Dr. Marc Hirsh here to be my doctor."

I can only imagine God smiling and saying, "Now you're getting it. Just wait to see how really thankful you're going to be for him when you see how I am going to use this doctor to change your life."

After that prayer, the rest is history, as they say. If you want to read the incredible story of Marc's spiritual journey to faith in Jesus as his Messiah, you'll have to read my first book, *When God & Cancer Meet*. But the short story of our "doctor-patient relationship" is that my family became close friends with Marc's family, and in 1996 he and his wife, Elizabeth, offered me a position in his office as a patient advocate providing emotional and spiritual care to cancer patients and their caregivers.

"Having a patient advocate makes so much sense that I wonder why we didn't do it sooner," he told me shortly after I started working with him, adding that he "can't imagine" practicing medicine without having someone in a position like mine.

I can't imagine what my life would be like *without* being a patient advocate. It's incredible to me what one small prayer of thankfulness has led to.

I'm wondering if you have found anything for which to be thankful in the midst of your circumstances. You or your loved one probably don't have a Messianic Jewish oncologist (if you do, I'd love to know!), but I believe there is something or someone for which you can say a prayer of thanks today. It may be just the prayer God wants to use to begin to bless your life.

The Old Testament prophet Habakkuk penned a wonderful example of thankfulness even when everything around him was going wrong:

> *Even though the fig trees have no blossoms,*
>   *and there are no grapes on the vines;*
> *even though the olive crop fails,*
>   *and the fields lie empty and barren;*
> *even though the flocks die in the fields,*
>   *and the cattle barns are empty,*
> *yet I will rejoice in the LORD!*
>   *I will be joyful in the God of my salvation!*
>   HABAKKUK 3:17-18

Go ahead, be thankful in all things—even when the hair follicles have no "blossoms" and even though your strength lies "empty and barren." Go ahead and rejoice in the Lord, because a prayer of thanksgiving can unleash the power of God in our lives in truly amazing ways.

Lord, give me the strength to do as it says in Romans 12:12: "Rejoice in hope, be patient in affliction, be faithful in prayer." Amen.

DAY 39
Anyone Can Beat Cancer

My friends Sandy and Ron Good are a fabulous example of "beating" cancer. Sandy was diagnosed with advanced ovarian cancer in June 2008, and Ron has been her biggest cheerleader and laughter "therapist" along the journey.

"Losing my hair was extremely difficult," Sandy recalls. "I knew it would come out and I thought I was prepared, but nothing prepares a lady to stare at her bald head. But I decided to look at the positive: showering was *so* easy. I didn't have to shampoo hair or shave my legs or under my arms.

"My husband said I was so fast in the shower that one day I would meet myself coming and going!"

Ron likes to explain that he was "Good" before he met Sandy, but she wasn't "Good" until she married him. I love Ron's quirky sense of humor, and I especially love that Sandy bakes wonderful goodies for our support group. (Just while I was typing this, she e-mailed me to say she has a Bundt cake, four dozen cookies, and a pan of brownies for tomorrow's meeting!)

And what I love most of all about this *really* Good couple is how they have refused to give in to cancer

and instead are beating it with supernatural strength
from God.

Would you be surprised if I told you Sandy's cancer
is not considered medically curable and doctors have
told her to expect it will take her life?

Perhaps you're wondering how she could "beat" cancer if she still has it in her body. Beating cancer is definitely about fighting this unseen enemy in an attempt
to be cured, and I would urge you to do that with
every breath in your body. But I also would urge you
to *enlarge* your view of what it means to beat cancer.

When I was first diagnosed with cancer, many well-
meaning friends told me, "You can beat this!" I know
those words were supposed to encourage me, but they
didn't. Instead, I thought, *Great! Now if I don't live, it's
my fault I didn't beat this because you said I could!*

I felt such pressure to "do everything right" to make
sure I beat cancer. I researched vitamins and herbs
and natural healing techniques. I listened to tapes by
alternative-medicine doctors promising cures for all.
I read stories of miraculous physical recoveries. But
nobody said beating cancer could be about more than
just a physical cure.

For quite a while, I was "beating" cancer—there was
no sign of it in my body—but at the same time, it was
beating me. It was controlling my mind, my attitude,

and my relationship with God. It was the first thing I thought about each day and the last thing each night. It was hard to enjoy holidays and special moments because I wondered if they would be my last. My prayer time consisted of nothing other than self-centered pleas for my personal healing.

But God gradually began to enlarge my picture of beating cancer as He spoke to my heart: "Whether you live or die from this is up to Me, but how you live is up to you."

The pressure was off. I would do my part to physically combat this cancer, but I would not judge whether I beat it by whether I was cured.

I would beat it *no matter what* because I would refuse to let it conquer me and control my life.

And by the grace of God I did, and I continue to do so more than two decades later.

I believe the real victory Sandy has over cancer is that she has triumphed over it in her mind and her spirit. She lives as a person who has cancer, but cancer does not have her. She is held in the palm of God's hand, not in the grip of a disease.

But beating cancer is not a one-moment or a one-day, once-and-for-all accomplishment.

☀ *Certainly, we beat cancer when we are declared in remission or cured.*

☀ *However, we also beat it moment by moment as we allow God, not cancer, to control our thoughts.*

☀ *We beat it hour by hour as we remember that God's power within us is greater than the cancer.*

☀ *And we beat it day by day as we trust in God's strength and not in cancer's weakness.*

The apostle Paul knew how to live in spite of his circumstances. He even wrote in chains from his jail cell:

Not that I speak from want, for I have learned to be content in whatever circumstances I am. I know how to get along with humble means, and I also know how to live in prosperity; in any and every circumstance I have learned the secret of being filled and going hungry, both of having abundance and suffering need. I can do all things through Him who strengthens me.
   PHILIPPIANS 4:11-13, NASB

☀ *Paul beat his circumstances.*

☀ *Sandy beat cancer.*

☀ *I beat cancer.*

☀ *You can beat cancer.*

Anyone can beat cancer because being victorious is much more than just being physically cured.

Lord, by Your strength today may my family and I beat cancer—body, mind, and spirit. In the victorious name of Jesus. Amen.

DAY 40
Praying without Words

It's pretty easy to thank God when everything's going well in your life. When you feel good. When you have your health.

It's a lot harder to praise Him when things—sometimes most things—are not going well. Before I was diagnosed with cancer, I always enjoyed singing in worship, praising God and thanking Him for all my wonderful blessings. Prayers came easily to my lips, especially prayers of thanksgiving, because I had a lot for which to be thankful. In fact, if you had told me there would come a time in my life when I wouldn't be able to pray, I would have laughed at the suggestion and insisted it could never happen.

But it did.

In those first dark days after my diagnosis, I literally couldn't pray. When I would read my Bible and then try to pray, the words simply would not form. Instead, tears rolled down my cheeks, sometimes just a trickle and sometimes turning into heavy sobs. The only thing I felt like I wanted to pray was a desperate cry for healing. What else was there to say?

And then I read a verse in the Bible—one I'm sure I'd read many times before, but it never had seemed that significant:

> *The Holy Spirit helps us in our distress. For we don't even know what we should pray for, nor how we should pray. But the Holy Spirit prays for us with groanings that cannot be expressed in words. And the Father who knows all hearts knows what the Spirit is saying, for the Spirit pleads for us believers in harmony with God's own will.*
> ROMANS 8:26-27

Two wonderful verses about how to pray when you feel you can't pray. They were right there in the Bible, sandwiched between Paul's discussion of suffering and his explanation of how we can be victorious even in difficult times! (Read the whole chapter and you'll see what I mean.)

It was okay that I felt I couldn't pray. The Holy Spirit would pray for me. He would take my "groans" that were too deep for words right to God Himself. And even better than that, the Spirit would know *what* to pray for me. He would pray according to God's will. I love how *The Message* renders Romans 8:26:

> *If we don't know how or what to pray, it doesn't matter. He does our praying in and for us, making prayer out of our wordless sighs, our aching groans.*

That's one amazing God! He knows that at the times we need Him most, we may not be able to express ourselves to Him, so He has His own Spirit do it for us! After I found that verse, I would often just sit, my hands on my lap, palms toward heaven, tears rolling down my cheeks . . . praying.

I never said a word. I couldn't even form cohesive thoughts in my mind, but I prayed. I didn't worry what or how to pray. I simply allowed God's Spirit to take my innermost thoughts, my deepest fears to God and pray for me.

In time I was able to pray again myself, but sometimes even now I still practice the kind of prayer I learned when I had no other way to pray.

Another amazing thing I learned about prayer during my cancer ordeal is that God has given us prayers we can pray when the pain is too deep.

I spent the entire six months of my chemo in the book of Psalms. I don't think I opened my Bible up anywhere except to the middle, where my eyes would fall upon a psalm that expressed my need to God.

I remember one day telling my husband how much the Psalms were blessing me as I dealt with the struggles of chemo treatments.

My surprised husband reminded me that in years past I had commented that those who wrote the sorrowful psalms seemed to be "a bunch of whiners."

"Well, now I'm a whiner too!" I explained.

It was true. For the first thirty-six years of my life, I had it really easy. A wonderful, loving home growing up; a good education; a great marriage; super children—nothing to whine about. Life had been so good that I had never needed God the way I did after I found out I had cancer.

Quite the contrary, the psalmists had plenty of

trouble in their lives, plenty of times they desperately needed God's help. So I read the Psalms. Day and night I read the Psalms as my prayers to God.

In you, LORD my God, I put my trust.
PSALM 25:1-2, NIV

I am worn out waiting for your rescue,
  but I have put my hope in your word.
PSALM 119:81

However you pray, your prayers are reaching the Father's ears. The Scriptures tell us that in Heaven there are "gold bowls filled with incense, which are the prayers of God's people" (Revelation 5:8; 8:3-4). Your prayer is a sweet fragrance to God. Here's one more from Psalm 119:116 you could pray today:

LORD, sustain me as you promised, that I may live! Do not let my hope be crushed. Amen.

(Just in case you don't have a Bible handy, I've included some of my favorite psalm prayers starting on page 219. Go ahead and fill up another bowlful in Heaven!)

DAY 41
Valley of Trouble

The other day I was reading in the book of Hosea about how God promised to "transform the Valley of Trouble into a gateway of hope" (2:15), and I thought of my friend Lauren.

His cancer journey has been an incredible roller coaster with hopes dashed one minute and unexpected new hopes found the next.

I hope your cancer journey or your loved one's is a much smoother, easier ride than Lauren's, but just in case you hit a bunch of bends in the road, I thought you should know his hope-filled story.

It all started in December 2006, when Lauren, then fifty-four, was diagnosed with a rare mantle cell non-Hodgkin's lymphoma. He began a course of chemo at nearby Hershey Medical Center, but never really got a good remission and restarted treatment in July 2008 when more tumors developed.

In November of that year, he walked his only daughter down the aisle (and unlike his wife, didn't have to worry about how his hair looked that day!). A couple of weeks later he headed back to Hershey for a stem cell transplant, because the chemo had not worked as well as hoped and he still had a lot of active disease.

Lauren received his stem cells from an anonymous donor because none of his family was a match for him. (The transplant involved Lauren receiving an intravenous lethal dose of chemo and then being "rescued" from death with a transfusion of the donor's healthy stem cells.)

Lauren survived the transplant, but some of the cancer also survived and started growing. The doctors tried a couple of new chemos, which didn't work, and then some radiation, which also failed to stop the tumors growing on his arm.

Finally in October 2009, the Hershey doctor said there was one more hope: a donor lymphocyte infusion. (Don't feel bad if you've never heard of it—Lauren hadn't either.) Basically, it involved putting some of the donor's white blood cells (lymphocytes) into him to see if they could recognize and destroy the cancer cells.

Lauren was the first to know the procedure was working.

"Within a week I could see the shrinkage in the tumors on my arm," he recalls.

A second dose was given, and the tumors disappeared. As I write, it's almost two years later, and

Lauren was just given another clean bill of health at Hershey. A few months ago he held his first grandson.

When I asked him how he managed to hang on through such a tough ordeal, he said, "My faith and the faith of others was what got me through. Many times I was about to throw in the towel, but my wife kept telling me 'Don't give up!'"

His wife, Joan, even gave him a quarter-sized medallion with the word *HOPE* emblazoned on it and told him to keep it in his pocket as a reminder that there still was hope for them.

That medallion is "still in there, and it's going to stay in there," says Lauren, who just last week learned the name of his German donor and can finally write him a heartfelt thank-you letter.

"I'm going to mail one of those [HOPE] coins to him so I can give back to him what he gave to me," Lauren adds.

He says there were times that he had doubts, worries, and fears, but found "when my faith was weak, the faith of others helped hold me up. The faith of other people, their prayers with me and the outpouring of support for me, gave me hope."

Recently, Lauren and his wife traveled West and stopped in Death Valley.

"I kept thinking about the verse, 'Yea, though I walk

through the valley of the shadow of death, I will fear no evil: for Thou art with me,'" recalls Lauren, quoting Psalm 23:4. "I knew I had come through that valley and He was with me."

As Lauren and I talked on the phone about this day's writing, he told me he was sitting and looking at his favorite picture in his home. It's a poster of a craggy mountaintop with this inscription underneath: "It's not the greatness of my faith that moves mountains, but my faith in the greatness of God."

☀ *Don't worry, my friend, if today your faith is not very big. Just be sure to put it all in a very big God.*

> *Great is the LORD! He is most worthy of praise!*
>   *No one can measure his greatness.*
>   PSALM 145:3

> *I will . . . transform the Valley of Trouble into*
> *a gateway of hope.*
>   HOSEA 2:15

Lord, I need You to walk with me through this dark valley. Help me not to give up, but to give in to You. I place my small faith in Your great power. Amen.

DAY 42
Unexpected Blessings

I'm always amazed when the discussion at my support group meetings turns to the *blessings* that have come through the survivors' cancer experiences. Somehow the words *blessing* and *cancer* in the same sentence just don't make sense.

I'm a very logical, rational person, and having colon cancer at the age of thirty-six made absolutely no sense to me. But as the years have gone by, I must admit that God has used this "senseless" experience to bring blessing in my life.

In May 1991, when I returned for my first checkup after six months of weekly chemo, I was the only person who wasn't there for a treatment that day. I knew I should feel happy that I had finished treatment, but I didn't. As I looked around that room of people in recliners, hooked up to poles with saline-solution bags, I was overcome with sadness. Some of them looked so thin and ill, and others looked so tired and afraid. I began to weep. I wanted to take away their pain, but I couldn't. I wanted to give them peace, but I couldn't.

Then God spoke to my heart: "But you know the One who can, and you can tell them about Me."

"But I just want to put all this behind me and go on with my life," I argued. "Besides, I don't want to hang around people with cancer. It will be depressing."

Finally, a few weeks later, like a pouting child, I gave in: "I'll do it, but I won't like it," I told Him.

I started the Cancer Prayer Support Group in October 1991 with four people. My intent was to have a one-hour, once-a-month meeting. *That shouldn't be too depressing*, I figured.

But almost immediately I could see that the people coming to the group needed more support than that. Not only that, but I found that I actually felt *better* after the meetings rather than worse. So we started meeting twice a month and have been doing so ever since. And guess what soon became a great source of joy in my life? The support group! As the months rolled by, I secretly began to pray that I would be able to quit my public relations job and volunteer with cancer patients.

In July 1995, on the fifth anniversary of my cancer surgery, I told our congregation how God had blessed me through my cancer experience—through my friends in the support group and through Marc and his wife, Elizabeth, who by then had become very close friends and prayer partners with my husband and me.

I concluded with this sentence: "Someday I hope I can quit my job and minister full-time, sharing God's peace and love with cancer patients."

I knew it was an unrealistic wish—there was no way financially that we could afford for me to quit my job and volunteer. But less than a year later, my prayer became a reality when Marc offered me a job in his office ministering to his patients' emotional and spiritual needs.

So since May 1, 1996, I have been a patient advocate, listening to patients' hopes and fears and praying that God will heal them physically, emotionally, and spiritually. I ask Him to bless each one, and I believe that He will.

In the year before my new job offer, I had been meditating on Ephesians 3:20, which speaks of our God "who is able to do immeasurably more than all we ask or imagine" (NIV).

There is no doubt in my mind that God has done far more in my life than I could ask or imagine, and I know that He can do that in your life too.

Do I think He's going to give you a job as a patient advocate for your oncologist? Probably not.

Do I think He is able to do something equally amazing in your life? You bet I do.

✹ *I can't tell you how, when, or where God will bring a*
   blessing through your trial of suffering. But I can tell
   you why—because His Word promises He will.

Romans 8:28 (NASB) says,

We know that God causes all things to work
together for good to those who love God, to those
who are called according to His purpose.

God will bring blessing through your trial because
you matter greatly to Him and He longs to show you
that. He may bless you with physical healing, or He
may bless you by healing you emotionally of some
deep-seated hurts. He may bless you spiritually with
the joy of knowing Him in a way you never have before.
Or He may bless others *through* you in unimaginable
ways.

My blessing from cancer is certainly *not* the one I
sought, but because God knows me and loves me, He
knew how to bless me.

He knows you. He loves you. He can bless you
through cancer . . . if you let Him decide the blessing.

Perhaps you would like to use part of Psalm 139 as
your prayer today:

*Lord, You go before me and follow me. You place Your
hand of blessing on my head. Such knowledge is too wonderful for me, too great for me to understand! I'm believing
that You can bring blessing through cancer, and I'm trusting
You to choose the blessing. Amen.*

DAY 43
The Thing with Feathers

I know I promised you that every patient story in this
book would have a happy ending, and I believe I'm
keeping my promise with my friend Carollynn's story,
although her final cancer cure came in Heaven and not
here on earth.

Personally, I think that someone who is diagnosed
with a brain tumor and given *no* chance of survival but
lives more than eight years cancer-free, then another
seven months after the tumor recurs, and then forever
in Heaven with her Savior *does* have a happy ending to
her story. (I hope you agree and keep reading.)

If you had asked Carollynn what gave her hope
throughout her cancer journey, she would have smiled
and answered "feathers."

She loved Emily Dickinson's poem "The Thing with Feathers," which begins:

> *"Hope" is the thing with feathers—*
> *That perches in the soul—*
> *And sings the tune without the words—*
> *And never stops—at all.*[32]

And when she was first diagnosed with cancer in 1995 at the age of forty-six, Carollynn stumbled upon a verse in the Bible that became her favorite:

> *He will cover you with his feathers.*
> *He will shelter you with his wings.*
> *His faithful promises are your armor and*
> *   protection.*
> PSALM 91:4

Even though medical doctors and treatments at that time gave her no hope of surviving more than a few months, this verse gave Carollynn incredible hope. It also started a real fascination with "feathers" and the number 914.

"Whenever I see a feather, it reminds me of God's protection for me," she told me shortly after moving to the area and joining my support group. "And I like to look for the number 914 on signs to remind me of God's constant care for me."

I had to chuckle when Carollynn's first grandchild was born on her birthday and weighed 9 pounds, 14 ounces! When Carollynn passed away just a few months later at 4:19 p.m., her husband, Ed, said he had to smile at what he felt was a last gift from Carollynn to remind him of her special verse.

"One final example of her fabulous humor," he wrote in an e-mail to friends and family.

Some of Carollynn's amazing life under God's wings was told in a children's book called *Sea Feather*, named after the first of many wild ponies she purchased on Chincoteague Island, Virginia, and donated to deserving children. More of her "feather-filled" life was shared in a video that aired on the television network *Animal Planet* in November 2003, just a month after her passing. (The nonprofit Feather Fund has been established to continue her work of donating wild ponies to children.)[33] When I see feathers today, they remind me of my beautiful friend Carollynn, but they also remind me of my God whose "wings" protect us even in the face of cancer.

Keep me as the apple of your eye;
*   hide me in the shadow of your wings.*
   PSALM 17:8, NIV

Let me live forever in your sanctuary,
*   safe beneath the shelter of your wings!*
    PSALM 61:4

Because you are my help,
*   I sing in the shadow of your wings.*
I cling to you;
*   your right hand upholds me.*
    PSALM 63:7-8, NIV

Of course, God the Father, who is Spirit, doesn't have real flesh-and-blood wings, but He is able to protect us by His awesome power.

Can you feel those "wings" over you—protecting you, shielding you, drawing you close? Have you trusted God enough to truly let Him cover you? He longs to do that for you.

Jesus said in Matthew 23:37,

How often I have wanted to gather your children
together as a hen protects her chicks beneath her
wings, but you wouldn't let me.

☀ **Please let God love you today. Let Him draw you close.**

My heart has heard you say, "Come and talk
  with me."
  And my heart responds, "LORD, I am coming."
  PSALM 27:8

Heavenly Father, thank You that You love us so much.
Thank You that Your loving arms are far bigger than any
cancer diagnosis or prognosis. Wrap my friend in that love
today. In Jesus' name. Amen.

DAY 44
Valley of Weeping

When I was taking chemo and attending the local hospital's cancer support group, a woman there shared that
her church was praying for her and she hadn't been sick
at all during her treatment.

Everyone in the group smiled and seemed to really
appreciate her story, but it ticked me off!

Why? Because my church and *lots* of churches were
praying for me, and I was sick all the time!

So I'm the last person who's going to *promise* you
that if you just pray, your or your loved one's treatment
will be a piece of cake. However, I do know plenty of
people who have basically waltzed through treatments

without any serious side effects. My friend Blaine had chemo and radiation for esophageal cancer and did so well he was even able to eat spicy chili with no problem. My friend Anne, an RN, never missed a day of work during the time she was bombarded with three chemos and a month of radiation for small-cell lung cancer back in 1994.

I hope and pray that your or your loved one's treatments go exceedingly well. The vast improvements in anti-nausea medicine since I was treated in 1990 are wonderful, and I can honestly say that the vast majority of patients in our office never get sick from chemo.

But just in case you or your loved one has a difficult time during treatment, I thought I should share about a friend for whom things didn't go so well. Before you stop reading, remember that it's a story of *hope* and it has a very happy ending!

Terry, a successful businessman, was diagnosed with tonsil cancer at the age of fifty-four. The diagnosis was a shock, and Terry admits to being filled with fear, especially of dying. He had his tonsils removed and then started thirty-five radiation treatments with some chemo added in.

"Gradually the eating just got worse and worse," Terry recalls. "At first I could eat chicken noodle soup, but then I had to switch to chicken and stars because the stars were smaller, and then I couldn't even eat anything but the broth."

The pounds kept falling off, and a feeding tube was inserted into his stomach so Terry could get the nutrition he so desperately needed. He was unable to work, and not surprisingly, depression set in.

Meanwhile, his wife, Pam, found her way to my cancer support group.

"Terry was too depressed to come with me, so I decided I would go by myself because I needed some support," Pam recalls.

Our group began praying for Terry to feel God's love for him and to reach out for His touch. It wasn't long before that prayer was answered.

"I remember I was really upset and wailing," Terry recalls. "I was so upset that Pam even called [my sister] Jackie and she called you. But then you called me and prayed for me on the phone. That really helped me."

Soon afterward Jackie shared the gospel with her brother, explaining how he could have his sins forgiven and be transformed by the power of God. Terry prayed with Jackie for that salvation, and my husband baptized him a few weeks later.

"I didn't have God in my life before," Terry says. "But after that, things changed. I started to attend church and put my whole situation in the Lord's hands."

As he prepares to celebrate his five-year cancer-free anniversary, Terry says he sees many blessings that have come from his difficult cancer journey.

"The biggest thing is being saved and turning to Christ," he explains. "And now being able to pray for people with cancer is really rewarding. It feels really good to encourage others and help them through their tough times."

There's a wonderful verse in the Bible that I think perfectly describes Terry and Pam's journey with cancer:

> When they walk through the Valley of Weeping,
>   it will become a place of refreshing springs.
>   The autumn rains will clothe it with blessings.
> PSALM 84:6

Are you in the Valley of Weeping today? Will you dare to believe that God can make it become a place of refreshing springs? That He can clothe you with blessings in spite of the trial you face today? Read His promise in Isaiah 43:2 from *The Message*:

> When you're in over your head, I'll be there with you.
>   When you're in rough waters, you will not go down.
>   When you're between a rock and a hard place,
>   it won't be a dead end.

God can make a way for you. Please let me pray for you as I did for Terry many years ago:

Dear Lord, it's so hard to walk through the valley and not see any way out. Please give my friend hope today that nothing is too difficult for You and that You can bring refreshing springs and even blessings from this trial. Give my friend the perseverance to hold on while waiting for that answer to prayer. In Jesus' name. Amen.

DAY 45
The Reason for Cancer

Everything happens for a reason.

Has anyone said that to you since your or your loved one's diagnosis? I'm wondering how it made you feel. I have to be honest and say that phrase usually annoys me. So if it's your favorite phrase in life and you love to say it or have people say it to you often, you might want to skip this day's reading.

Well, because you're still reading I have to believe it's for a reason (☺), and I'm praying God uses these words to give you hope today as we wonder together what's the "reason" for cancer.

I'm not sure who should get the original credit for

that phrase: "Everything happens for a reason." I've seen it attributed to Marilyn Monroe and Oprah Winfrey, and I'm sure many other famous and not-so-famous people have said it often. I remember using it myself when I was a new Christian back in college and someone stole my wallet right out of my purse in the checkout line at the campus bookstore. I was terribly distraught and remarked to my friend Vince, "I know everything happens for a reason, but I can't figure out what God is trying to teach me through this."

To which Vince replied, "I'll tell you the reason this happened—someone sinned and stole your wallet!"

I liked that explanation. I quit agonizing over some spiritual lesson God was trying to teach me. Oh, I definitely learned things from the incident—like closing up my purse faster and trusting God for the money I'd lost—but I stopped imagining that every single thing that happened to me throughout the day was orchestrated by God for a divine reason that I had to figure out.

The phrase "everything happens for a reason" probably has multiple meanings to the many folks who utter it. But the word *reason* by definition means there is an explanation, a justification or rational grounds for what's occurring. What's implied is there is a *good* reason behind every single thing that occurs. I'm just not sure that fits life here on earth.

What's the explanation for babies with cancer?

What's the justification for a married couple both having cancer at the same time?

What's the rational grounds for a young parent dying of cancer?

Scientists will tell you that the DNA mutations that cause cancer are influenced by many factors, including genetics, environment, and lifestyle.

If you can discover the physical reason(s) you or your loved one got cancer, that knowledge may help you make choices that reduce the chance the cancer will come back or help family members prevent having to face the disease themselves. Personally, I had absolutely no known risk factors for getting colorectal cancer, so I couldn't really make any lifestyle changes. I did have genetic testing for Lynch Syndrome, which detects inherited mutations for colorectal cancer, but I did not have any of the known variations.

I honestly never figured out the reason I got cancer, but whatever it was, I knew that reason did not have the final say in my life.

Remember Joseph, the young man in the Old Testament with the coat of many colors? His jealous brothers sold him into slavery, but he became a powerful person in Pharaoh's court and eventually saved their lives. When his brothers finally asked for forgiveness for their evil actions, Joseph replied, "You intended to harm me, but God intended it all for good" (Genesis 50:20).

☀ *I don't know why this ugly disease of cancer has "intended" to harm you, but I do know God can "intend" it for good.*

We know that God causes everything to work together for the good of those who love God and are called according to his purpose for them.
ROMANS 8:28

Please notice this is a conditional promise. The working-together-for-good only happens to people who "love God" and are "called according to his purpose."

The very next verse explains what that means. It says God "chose them to become like his Son." That's our purpose in life: to become more like Jesus. Then and *only* then can we be assured that everything that happens to us—even cancer—will be used by God for good.

Whatever the reason cancer has intruded into your life, here is my prayer for you today from Philippians 1:9-11:

I pray that your love will overflow more and more, and that you will keep on growing in knowledge and under-standing. For I want you to understand what really matters, so that you may live pure and blameless lives until the day of Christ's return. May you always be filled with the fruit of your salvation—the righteous character produced in your life by Jesus Christ—for this will bring much glory and praise to God. Amen.

P.S. Thanks for reading this today—I *do* believe it happened for a good reason!

DAY 46
ABCs of Trials

So if God can work all things together for good, does that mean in our lifetime we will see that promise come true?

Maybe, maybe not.

I consider myself extremely fortunate that God has allowed me to see firsthand how He has used my cancer diagnosis for good by giving me a worldwide ministry to cancer patients and their caregivers. However, I'm very aware that many others are still waiting to see that promise come true in their lives.

It's one thing to know that someday—eventually—God will bring good from your bad situation; it's another thing to have to live in that situation day by day. In those early, confusing post-diagnosis days, I had to come to terms with the fact that I didn't have the whole picture of what God was doing in and through my life.

Now we see things imperfectly as in a poor mirror, but then we will see everything with perfect clarity. All that I know now is partial and incomplete, but then I will know everything completely, just as God knows me now.
    1 CORINTHIANS 13:12

Our view from inside a cancer-storm is limited and distorted. We often cannot see how what is happening could ever possibly be used as part of God's good plan for our lives. We don't have the big picture.

But accepting that we don't have the whole picture is not very comforting unless we also realize that the One who *does* is the One who loves us greatly.

Some years ago our youngest daughter, Lindsey, who had just graduated from college (and as the daughter most like me, butted heads with me the most as a teenager), wrote me a Mother's Day note that said in part,

"I didn't always agree or understand when you said no to me, but I never doubted that you loved me."

That's what it means to trust. We choose never to doubt that God loves us even if we don't always agree or understand when He answers no to our prayers.

However, just knowing these two truths—that we don't have the whole picture and a loving God does—is not enough. We have to continue to walk by faith and not by sight. I'll be the first to admit that is not an easy task. Even if we're not from Missouri, we humans tend to be "show me" people. We want to see *first* and then believe. I am an extremely skeptical person (which makes me a great newspaper reporter but an annoying wife), and I *always* want the facts, the explanation, and the logic *before* I'll agree with just about anything.

But the Word of God, my compass in life and especially in the storms, tells me that as believers we are different from others in this world because "we live by faith, not by sight."[34] Or as another translation puts it, "That is why we live by believing and not by seeing."[35]

I must constantly remind myself that I don't need to see it all because God sees it all from the beginning of history to the end of time. As one writer explains:

> Because we see only this sliver of time, we
> tend to view all of time through the same

narrow and ill-fitting glasses. We forget that
God is not bound by time. He exists outside
of its minutes and millennia.[36]

He and only He has the big picture. We move
ahead not knowing for sure how it all will work out,
but believing He does and will guide our way. I don't
know how to say it any other way than we simply *walk
by faith.*

*Faith is confidence in what we hope for and
assurance about what we do not see.*
  HEBREWS 11:1, NIV

*Let us run with endurance the race God has
set before us. We do this by keeping our eyes
on Jesus, the champion who initiates and
perfects our faith.*
  HEBREWS 12:1-2

With our eyes on Jesus, we can continue to walk by
faith and not by sight. God's Word promises that He is
able even if we are not. We don't have to pull ourselves
up; His strength will hold us up. We don't have to just
put on a happy face; His peace will fill us up.

The LORD gives his people strength.
  The LORD blesses them with peace.
  PSALM 29:11

Remember the ABCs of trials: **A**ccept that you don't have the whole picture; **B**elieve a loving God does; and **C**ontinue on by faith and not by sight.

Lord, help me to keep my eyes on You and not on the storm around me. Increase my faith so that I can walk boldly in it as I trust You for each day. In Jesus' name. Amen.

DAY 47
Treasures in Darkness

I wish you could visit my Cancer Prayer Support Groups and meet the incredible survivors there.

I'd introduce you to Joan and Deb, both of whom have been cured of colorectal cancer despite its having spread to the liver. And you could meet our "star" colorectal survivor, Grace, whose cancer was diagnosed in 2002, spread to her liver in 2003, and then to an ovary in 2004. She's a beautiful lady now in her eighties, and tests continue to show her to be cancer-free!

And if he hadn't moved away, I'd introduce you

to Jason, whom I wrote about in my second book, *Finding the Light in Cancer's Shadow*. He was originally diagnosed with testicular cancer in 1995, and it spread to his spine in 2002, temporarily paralyzing him from the waist down. He's been off treatment for eight years, finished his master's degree, plays basketball, and fathered fraternal twins almost three years ago!

And I would love for you to meet Nancy, a six-year survivor of incurable liver cancer. Meetings are always better when she's there—partly because she's a wonderful baker (she brought *four* fresh strawberry pies to one meeting last summer), but mostly because she's just an awesome person.

Nancy originally was told in January 2005 that she had a "very aggressive" liver cancer and there wasn't anything anyone could do for her.

"If you have anything you want to do, you should do it," the doctor told her, adding that she probably would die within a month.

But about two weeks later, she got a call from another physician who said she had been misdiagnosed. It indeed was a rare, untreatable liver cancer, but a *slow-growing* one, which probably would not take her life.

With that good news, Nancy figured the hard part of her cancer journey was over, but she was very wrong.

One of her doctors suggested a new, oral chemo-therapy, which just might slow the cancer's growth, and Nancy agreed to give it a try. Unfortunately, one of the drug's side effects was severe depression.

"When I would wake up in the morning, I thought I couldn't get out of bed," Nancy recalls. "Any desire to do anything at all was gone. I would just sit and cry."

Nancy, of course, stopped the drug, but the depression lasted for *eighteen months*.

"I felt terribly alone even in a roomful of people," she recalls. "It was the most horrible feeling I've ever had."

I've never experienced that kind of depression, but I believe Nancy when she says it was "worse than being told I had cancer or that I was going to die."

So why am I telling you this story in a book about hope? Because Nancy got through her depression and is back to her bubbly self, and I want you to know that you and your loved one *can* survive depression if it should rear its ugly head in your lives.

Whenever a newcomer joins our support group and is struggling with depression, I want that person to meet Nancy because she's been there, done that. And most of all, I want them to hear what Nancy discovered during her ordeal.

"I learned that God is faithful," she says. "I always believed that, but not to the extent I do now."

"Even though I couldn't feel close to God then, I always sensed He was there," she says. "When I prayed to die in my sleep, the Holy Spirit was there with me, whispering, 'It's going to be OK—it's not over yet.' God was always there."

I will give you treasures hidden in the darkness—
secret riches.
I will do this so you may know that I am the LORD,
the God of Israel, the one who calls you by name.
ISAIAH 45:3

Nancy's path is not one she ever would have chosen for herself, but she wholeheartedly agrees that the Lord gave her treasures that were hidden in the darkness of depression. Now she eagerly shares those "secret riches" with those she meets who are struggling with their own despondent times.

"When I was down, just a teeny bit of hope helped me," Nancy remembers. "If I can give that to anyone, I'd be happy."

I always feel more hopeful when I talk to Nancy, as the love and light of God shine through her. She and her incredibly supportive husband, Tom, recently celebrated their fiftieth wedding anniversary by taking a trip to Belize—not as relaxing tourists, but to work at the orphanage they helped build.

"I just want to give back," Nancy explains. "I think that's why God left me here."

Father, I pray for anyone reading this today who is struggling with depression or any other dark cloud of discouragement. I pray that they will trust that You are faithful and will see them through. And I pray that one day they can look back and see the treasures You have brought to light through this time. In Jesus' name. Amen.

DAY 48
Everlasting Hope

What are you wishing for today?

A cure? A long remission? A successful surgery? A not-too-toxic treatment? More energy? Less pain?

And on what or whom are you pinning those hopes?

I've seen people put their hope in all sorts of things— vitamins, nutritional supplements, macrobiotic diets, and even coffee enemas. (I know one patient who completely depleted her body of electrolytes because of this daily cup of joe!) Some people put their hope in their doctor and his or her abilities. Some people feel they have no hope. Maybe some physician has even told you there *is* no hope.

When I was going through my treatments for cancer and then living with the reality that I had maybe a 40-percent chance of surviving cancer, many people asked me, "How do you do it?" The answer was that I had hope. Nothing about my cancer made any sense to me.

Why should I, a young, healthy person have cancer?

Why should my husband have to face the possibility of being widowed again?

Why should my little girls fear growing up without their mother?

None of it made sense.

Only one thing did make sense, and that was knowing this life is not all there is because I had an eternal hope. Think about it . . . even if you or your loved one survive cancer, you still will die someday. I know people who have survived cancer only to be cut down suddenly by heart attacks, and I know family members of cancer patients who unexpectedly passed away while the patients unexpectedly survived their cancer. No matter how many times we get healed on this earth, one day the healing will cease here. And that's why we all need an eternal hope.

You see, we all have the same terminal sickness. It's

congenital because we're all born with it. The symptoms aren't always obvious, but they appear throughout life in the bad things we say and do, and in the good things we fail to say and do.

The Bible explains this worldwide epidemic in Romans 3:23: "Everyone has sinned; we all fall short of God's glorious standard." And the end result of sin is clearly spelled out in Romans 6:23: "The wages of sin is death."

So sin is the diagnosis for all of us, and terminal is the prognosis for everyone.

Don't be fooled into thinking you don't have it. Just like cancer, it's a very sneaky condition, and you can look perfectly fine on the outside while you're dying on the inside.

But I have good news—there is a cure. It's extremely expensive, but the entire cost has been paid up front for us.

> *God paid a ransom to save you. . . . It was the precious blood of Christ.*
> 1 PETER 1:18-19

If you've never experienced the cure for your sin sickness, you can right now. You must agree with God's diagnosis that you are a sinner and desire to get a new prognosis by accepting His gift of eternal life. If you do, Jesus will forgive your sins, lead your life, and one day take you to your real home in Heaven.

> *If I go and prepare a place for you, I will come back and take you to be with me that you also may be where I am. . . . I am the way and the truth and the life. No one comes to the Father except through me.*
> JOHN 14:3, 6, NIV

I hope and pray that you and your loved ones live long, healthy, happy lives and that cancer soon becomes a distant memory. But while that prayer is sincere, it also is a shortsighted prayer. I don't just care about what happens to your bodies and minds here on earth, but I care about what happens to your souls after you leave this earth.

And that's why I pray that you and your loved ones have an eternal hope—an ultimate hope—a hope that transcends all other hopes.

> *We wait for the blessed hope—the appearing of the glory of our great God and Savior, Jesus Christ, who gave himself for us to redeem us.*
> TITUS 2:13-14, NIV

This hope is a strong and trustworthy anchor for our souls.
  HEBREWS 6:19

I have had that blessed hope since I put my trust in Jesus in 1972 while a student at the Ohio State University. That is why after my diagnosis, I knew where I was going to spend eternity if I was to die from cancer (or anything else). I knew life was not being fair to me, but God would be. He had provided a way for me to get to Heaven—where Scripture promises no more tears, no more sickness, and no more dying (Revelation 21:4). I was not getting shortchanged if I died young, because this life is not all there is. Now that made sense . . . and gave me hope.

And so, Lord, where do I put my hope? My only hope is in you.
  PSALM 39:7

Dear God, my prayer today is that each person reading this is looking to You not just for earthly hopes, but for an eternal hope. May each one trust in You for the forgiveness of sins and accept Your free gift of everlasting life. Thank You for the blessed hope that Jesus will come back one day and take each of us believers home. I pray in His name. Amen.

DAY 49
Waste Not, Want Not

"Don't waste your cancer."

Those are the words penned by author-pastor John Piper on the eve of his surgery for prostate cancer in 2006. Our Cancer Prayer Support Group often spends a meeting discussing one of Piper's ten ways we can "waste" cancer by allowing it—instead of God—to be foremost in our lives. (You can read his wonderful essay at www.desiringgod.org.) Many in our group have embraced Piper's admonition and often will remark, "I don't want to waste this cancer."

Probably the cancer survivor who most often expresses that sentiment is my friend Bert, diagnosed in December 2003 with Stage 4 prostate cancer at the age of sixty-eight.

Bert's cancer was not operable, so he underwent eight weeks of radiation and eighteen months of hormone shots to try to slow its course. The radiation went fairly well, but the shots, which "turned off" his male hormones gave him severe hot flashes.

"That gave me a greater appreciation of what women go through in menopause, and I sure don't want to go through childbirth!" Bert admits with a smile.

Because Bert's father and grandfather both had faced cancer, he wasn't particularly stunned to get his diagnosis.

"I was surprised and concerned, but I had a peace about it," he recalls. "I remember thinking that I could go home and feel sorry for myself—but I would still have cancer—or I could use it to show people that I'm not afraid to die. I've decided I will use cancer to share and encourage other people."

☀ *Don't waste your cancer.*

That's the decision Bert made many years ago. Since then, his yearly PSA readings are in the normal range as he continues to be in complete remission from the cancer. But he has been told by doctors to expect it to come back at some point.

"Can it come back? Yeah," he says. "Am I afraid of that? No."

Bert says his peace about his uncertain future comes from the fact that he is a "Christ-follower."

"I love to explain to people what that means," he adds. "I like to ask people, 'Where is your hope?' And I like to share with them that my hope is in following Christ."

I am so glad that Bert decided not to waste his cancer.

I can't begin to tell you all the folks in our support group he has encouraged in their cancer fight, as well as many others in his church and community.

I'd like to think I haven't wasted my cancer either. I'll admit I initially was rather reluctant (okay, *very* reluctant) to minister to cancer patients and their caregivers. But the more I reached out to hurting people, the more I got blessed too. I realized I couldn't go back and change my diagnosis, my treatment, or even my prognosis, but I could make sure that all the pain I endured was not wasted. I had suffered on my cancer journey, but I also had been comforted by God, and I could share that truth with others. As the apostle Paul explains in 2 Corinthians 1:3-4:

> *God is our merciful Father and the source of all comfort. He comforts us in all our troubles so that we can comfort others. When they are troubled, we will be able to give them the same comfort God has given us.*

Whatever you and your family have suffered—whatever hardship still lies ahead for you—will you ask God today to help you not waste it?

Piper further explains in his essay how a crisis can become an opportunity:

> Christians are never anywhere by divine accident. There are reasons for why we wind up where we do. Consider what Jesus said about painful, unplanned circumstances: "They will lay their hands on you and persecute you, delivering you up to the synagogues and prisons, and you will be brought before kings and governors for my name's sake. This will be your opportunity to bear witness." (Luke 21:12-13). So it is with cancer. This will be an opportunity to bear witness. Christ is infinitely worthy. Here is a golden opportunity to show that he is worth more than life. Don't waste it.[37]

Heavenly Father, I wish I didn't have to face cancer, but because I do, I'm asking You to help me not to waste it. Please take these painful, unplanned circumstances and turn them into an opportunity for me to show others that You are worth more than life itself. In Jesus' name I pray. Amen.

DAY 50
Living Free of Cancer

Would you believe that I've prayed for you even though I probably will never know your name? I have. Many times.

I prayed God would direct people to pick up this book so He might encourage them. I prayed that even if *we* never meet, you still would meet God and that *He* would meet your deepest needs.

It's the same thing I prayed for my other books, and I've heard many incredible stories of how this came true. Some people have even tracked me down and written or called to tell me amazing things that happened when they were reading them. A handful of readers even drove hours to visit my Cancer Prayer Support Group just to see if we really laugh as much as I said we did!

I'd love to get a bunch of these survivors together and have a radio program where anyone who has gotten good test results or had successful surgery could call in and share their encouraging stories. You know, kind of a spin-off of the Dave Ramsey radio talk show where he preaches a message of living debt-free and when people reach that coveted pinnacle, they call in and scream on air at the top of their lungs, "I'm DEBT-FREE!"

Well, on my show, cancer patients would call in and holler, "I'm CANCER-FREE!"

I think a cancer-free survivors' show would be a great program to tune into every day!

But my ultimate hope and my prayer is that *all* of us cancer survivors and our loved ones could call up and proclaim, "I'm free of cancer!" Not just free of it in our bodies, but free of it in our minds and our spirits.

Thank you for spending these fifty days with me. I know that everyone needs *more than* just fifty days of hope. In fact, there's an old proverb that says you can live three weeks without food, three days without water, three minutes without air, but only three seconds without hope. You're going to need hope every single day of your remaining cancer journey. I won't be with you each day (unless you read my other books!). But don't worry; my words are not your source of hope. They only serve to point you to the truth.

His name will be the hope
   of all the world.
   MATTHEW 12:21

That name that is above all names is the name of Jesus. He is the best hope for cancer survivors, their loved ones, and truly for the whole world.

> *Rejoice in our confident hope. Be patient in trouble, and keep on praying.*
> ROMANS 12:12

In the Lord you can find as many days of hope as you need. You will never run out of hope.

Ask Him and trust Him to keep your mind, your heart, and your soul free of cancer—whether or not your body is. Then you will be able to say with me:

☀ *Cancer does not occupy my mind.*

It is seized with God's perfect peace.

☀ *Cancer has no place in my heart.*

It is filled with God's awesome love.

☀ *Cancer cannot touch my soul.*

It is saved by God's amazing grace.

☀ *I am free of cancer.*

My prayer for you today—and every single day God gives you—is from Romans 15:13:

I pray that God, the source of hope, will fill you completely with joy and peace because you trust in Him. Then you will overflow with confident hope through the power of the Holy Spirit. I pray this in the hope-filled name of Jesus. Amen.

Fear Not!

I prayed to the LORD, and he answered me.
  He freed me from all my fears.
    PSALM 34:4

He grants the desires of those who fear him;
  he hears their cries for help and rescues them.
    PSALM 145:19

The LORD is for me, so I will have no fear.
  What can mere people do to me?
    PSALM 118:6

You can go to bed without fear;
  you will lie down and sleep soundly.
    PROVERBS 3:24

God has not given us a spirit of fear and timidity,
but of power, love, and self-discipline.
    2 TIMOTHY 1:7

I (Paul) am convinced that nothing can ever separate
us from God's love. Neither death nor life, neither
angels nor demons, neither our fears for today nor
our worries about tomorrow—not even the powers
of hell can separate us from God's love.
    ROMANS 8:38

Waiting More (and Despising It Less)

Wait patiently for the LORD.
   Be brave and courageous.
   Yes, wait patiently for the LORD.
      PSALM 27:14

LORD, I wait for you;
   you will answer, Lord my God.
      PSALM 38:15, NIV

I wait for the LORD, my whole being waits,
   and in his word I put my hope.
      PSALM 130:5, NIV

Let all that I am wait quietly before God,
   for my hope is in him.
      PSALM 62:5

As for me, I watch in hope for the LORD,
   I wait for God my Savior;
   my God will hear me.
      MICAH 7:7, NIV

The LORD must wait for you to come to him
   so he can show you his love and compassion
For the LORD is a faithful God.
   Blessed are those who wait for his help.
      ISAIAH 30:18

Since the world began,
    no ear has heard
and no eye has seen a God like you,
    who works for those who wait for him!
        ISAIAH 64:4

We wait in hope for the LORD;
    he is our help and our shield.
In him our hearts rejoice,
    for we trust in his holy name.
May your unfailing love be with us, LORD,
    even as we put our hope in you.
        PSALM 33:20-22, NIV

When Worries Make You Sweat the Small (and Big) Stuff

Worry weighs a person down;
    an encouraging word cheers a person up.

    PROVERBS 12:25

Refuse to worry, and keep your body healthy.

    ECCLESIASTES 11:10

If God cares so wonderfully for wildflowers that are here today and thrown into the fire tomorrow, he will certainly care for you. Why do you have so little faith? So don't worry about these things, saying, "What will we eat? What will we drink? What will we wear?" These things dominate the thoughts of unbelievers, but your heavenly Father already knows all your needs.

    MATTHEW 6:30-32

Can all your worries add a single moment to your life? And if worry can't accomplish a little thing like that, what's the use of worrying over bigger things?

    LUKE 12:25-26

Don't worry about tomorrow, for tomorrow will bring its own worries. Today's trouble is enough for today.

    MATTHEW 6:34

Healing Thoughts

Have compassion on me, LORD, for I am weak.
　　Heal me, LORD, for my bones are in agony.
　　　　PSALM 6:2

O LORD my God, I cried to you for help,
　　and you restored my health.
　　　　PSALM 30:2

Let all that I am praise the LORD;
　　may I never forget the good things he does for me.
He forgives all my sins
　　and heals all my diseases.
　　　　PSALM 103:2-3

"LORD, help!" they cried in their trouble,
　　and he saved them from their distress.
He sent out his word and healed them,
　　snatching them from the door of death.
　　　　PSALM 107:19-20

Don't be impressed with your own wisdom.
　　Instead, fear the LORD and turn away from evil.
Then you will have healing for your body
　　and strength for your bones.
　　　　PROVERBS 3:7-8

A cheerful look brings joy to the heart;
   good news makes for good health.
      PROVERBS 15:30

A cheerful heart is good medicine,
   but a broken spirit saps a person's strength.
      PROVERBS 17:22

My child, pay attention to what I say.
   Listen carefully to my words.
Don't lose sight of them.
   Let them penetrate deep into your heart,
for they bring life to those who find them,
   and healing to their whole body.
      PROVERBS 4:20-22

Give Peace a Chance

May the LORD show you his favor
    and give you his peace.
        NUMBERS 6:26

In peace I will lie down and sleep,
    for you alone, O LORD, will keep me safe.
        PSALM 4:8

I listen carefully to what God the LORD is saying,
    for he speaks peace to his faithful people.
    But let them not return to their foolish ways.
        PSALM 85:8

A peaceful heart leads to a healthy body;
    jealousy is like cancer in the bones.
        PROVERBS 14:30

You will keep in perfect peace
    all who trust in you,
    all whose thoughts are fixed on you!
        ISAIAH 26:3

Because of God's tender mercy,
    the morning light from heaven is about to break
        upon us,

to give light to those who sit in darkness and in the
    shadow of death,
  and to guide us to the path of peace.
    LUKE 1:78-79

Jesus said:

I am leaving you with a gift—peace of mind and
heart. And the peace I give is a gift the world cannot
give. So don't be troubled or afraid.
    JOHN 14:27

I have told you all this so that you may have peace
in me. Here on earth you will have many trials and
sorrows. But take heart, because I have overcome
the world.
    JOHN 16:33

The apostle Paul said:

Letting your sinful nature control your mind leads to
death. But letting the Spirit control your mind leads
to life and peace.
    ROMANS 8:6

I pray that God, the source of hope, will fill you
completely with joy and peace because you trust in
him. Then you will overflow with confident hope
through the power of the Holy Spirit.

    ROMANS 15:13

Let the peace that comes from Christ rule in your
hearts. For as members of one body you are called
to live in peace. And always be thankful.

    COLOSSIANS 3:15

May the Lord of peace himself give you his peace
at all times and in every situation. The Lord be with
you all.

    2 THESSALONIANS 3:16

Psalm Prayers

For "whiners" like me and anyone else wanting to cry out to God. Whenever I came to the word *enemy* or *enemies*, I substituted *cancer* because it was my biggest enemy!

O Lord, how long will you forget me? Forever?
   How long will you look the other way?
How long must I struggle with anguish in my soul,
   with sorrow in my heart every day?
   How long will my enemy have the upper hand?

Turn and answer me, O Lord my God!
   Restore the sparkle to my eyes, or I will die.
Don't let my enemies gloat, saying, "We have
     defeated him!"
   Don't let them rejoice at my downfall.
But I trust in your unfailing love.
   I will rejoice because you have rescued me.
I will sing to the Lord
   because he is good to me.

    Psalm 13

Lord, hear my prayer!
  Listen to my plea!
Don't turn away from me
  in my time of distress.
Bend down to listen,
  and answer me quickly when I call to you.
For my days disappear like smoke,
  and my bones burn like red-hot coals.
My heart is sick, withered like grass,
  and I have lost my appetite.
Because of my groaning,
  I am reduced to skin and bones. . . .
He broke my strength in midlife,
  cutting short my days.
But I cried to him, "O my God, who lives forever,
  don't take my life while I am so young!

  Psalm 102:1-5, 23-24

Save me, O God,
  for the floodwaters are up to my neck.
Deeper and deeper I sink into the mire;
  I can't find a foothold.
I am in deep water,

and the floods overwhelm me.
I am exhausted from crying for help;
   my throat is parched.
My eyes are swollen with weeping,
   waiting for my God to help me. . . .
Answer my prayers, O Lord,
   for your unfailing love is wonderful.
Take care of me,
   for your mercy is so plentiful.
Don't hide from your servant;
   answer me quickly, for I am in deep trouble!
Come and redeem me;
   free me from my enemies.

    Psalm 69:1-3, 16-18

Bend down, O Lord, and hear my prayer;
   answer me, for I need your help.
Protect me, for I am devoted to you.
   Save me, for I serve you and trust you.
   You are my God.
Be merciful to me, O Lord,
   for I am calling on you constantly.
Give me happiness, O Lord,

for I give myself to you.
O Lord, you are so good, so ready to forgive,
    so full of unfailing love for all who ask for your
        help.
Listen closely to my prayer, O LORD;
    hear my urgent cry.
I will call to you whenever I'm in trouble,
    and you will answer me.
        PSALM 86:1-7

I cry out to the LORD;
    I plead for the LORD's mercy.
I pour out my complaints before him
    and tell him all my troubles.
When I am overwhelmed,
    you alone know the way I should turn.
Wherever I go,
    my enemies have set traps for me.
I look for someone to come and help me,
    but no one gives me a passing thought!
No one will help me;
    no one cares a bit what happens to me.
Then I pray to you, O LORD.

I say, "You are my place of refuge.
    You are all I really want in life."
 PSALM 142:1-5

The LORD is my light and my salvation—
    so why should I be afraid?
The LORD is my fortress, protecting me from danger,
    so why should I tremble?
When evil people come to devour me,
    when my enemies and foes attack me,
    they will stumble and fall.
Though a mighty army surrounds me,
    my heart will not be afraid.
Even if I am attacked,
    I will remain confident.
The one thing I ask of the LORD—
    the thing I seek most—
is to live in the house of the LORD all the days
        of my life,
    delighting in the LORD's perfections
    and meditating in his Temple.
 PSALM 27:1-4

I love you, LORD;
　　you are my strength.
The LORD is my rock, my fortress, and my savior;
　　my God is my rock, in whom I find protection.
He is my shield, the power that saves me,
　　and my place of safety.
I called on the LORD, who is worthy of praise,
　　and he saved me from my enemies.

The ropes of death entangled me;
　　floods of destruction swept over me.
The grave wrapped its ropes around me;
　　death laid a trap in my path.
But in my distress I cried out to the LORD;
　　yes, I prayed to my God for help.
He heard me from his sanctuary;
　　my cry to him reached his ears.

　　PSALM 18:1-6

I look up to the mountains—
　　does my help come from there?

My help comes from the LORD,
   who made heaven and earth!

He will not let you stumble;
   the one who watches over you will not slumber.
Indeed, he who watches over Israel
   never slumbers or sleeps.

The LORD himself watches over you!
   The LORD stands beside you as your protective
     shade.
The sun will not harm you by day,
   nor the moon at night.

The LORD keeps you from all harm
   and watches over your life.
The LORD keeps watch over you as you come and go,
   both now and forever.

   PSALM 121

Notes

1. Devotional writings of Max Lucado, found in *Grace for the Moment Daily Bible*, New Century Version (Nashville: Thomas Nelson, 2006), 20.

2. National Cancer Institute, The SEER Cancer Statistics Review (CSR), 1975–2008, http://seer.cancer.gov /csr/1975_2008/results_merged/topic_survival.pdf.

3. M. Scott Peck, *Further Along the Road Less Traveled* (New York: Touchstone, 1993), 23.

4. Susan Lenzkes, *When Life Takes What Matters*, quoted by Anne Cetas, *Our Daily Bread*, June 25, 2007, http://odb .org/2007/06/25/reach-for/.

5. Francis S. Collins, *The Language of God: A Scientist Presents Evidence for Belief* (New York: Simon & Schuster, 2007), 1.

6. Ibid., 3.

7. Ibid., 233.

8. Philip Yancey, *Disappointment with God* (Grand Rapids: Zondervan, 1988), 182–184.

9. NIV

10. THE MESSAGE

11. NLT

12. Henry T. Blackaby and Richard Blackaby, *Experiencing God Day by Day Devotional* (Nashville: Broadman & Holman, 1998), 94. The story of the Israelites being led by God with a cloud and a pillar of fire is found in Exodus 13:21.

13. Ibid.

14. "NTSB: Pilot Disorientation Led to Fatal JFK Jr. Crash,"
    CNN.com, July 6, 2000, http://www.ntsb.gov/news
    /2000/000706.htm.

15. Max Lucado, *When God Whispers Your Name* (Nashville:
    Thomas Nelson, 2009), 214.

16. Rick Warren, *The Purpose Driven Life* (Grand Rapids:
    Zondervan, 2002), 202.

17. Norman Cousins, *Head First: The Biology of Hope and the
    Healing Power of the Human Spirit* (New York: Penguin,
    1990), 239.

18. Charles L. Allen, *All Things Are Possible through Prayer*
    (Old Tappan, NJ: Revell, 2003), 51.

19. Lance Armstrong, *It's Not about the Bike: My Journey Back
    to Life* (New York: G. F. Putnam's Sons, 2001), 112.

20. Corrie ten Boom, *The Hiding Place* (Grand Rapids:
    Chosen Books, 1984), 44.

21. Rick Warren, *The Purpose Driven Life* (Grand Rapids:
    Zondervan, 2002), 69.

22. Jimmie Holland and Sheldon Lewis, *The Human Side
    of Cancer: Living with Hope, Coping with Uncertainty*
    (New York: HarperCollins, 2001), 14.

23. Ibid., 30–31.

24. Mike Dellosso, *The Hunted* (Lake Mary, FL: Realms,
    2008). www.mikedellosso.com.

25. David Biebel, *If God Is So Good, Why Do I Hurt So Bad?*
    (Grand Rapids: Revell, 1989), 15.

26. NASB

27. Young's Literal Translation

28. AMP

29. CEV

30. Max Lucado, *In the Grip of Grace* (Nashville: Thomas Nelson, 2009), 180.

31. Charles R. Swindoll, *Strengthening Your Grip* (Nashville: W Publishing Group, 1982), 206–207. Used by permission of Insight for Living (the Bible-teaching ministry of Charles R. Swindoll), Plano, TX 75025. All rights reserved.

32. Emily Dickinson, found in *The Complete Poems of Emily Dickinson*, ed. Thomas H. Johnson (New York: Little Brown, 1961), 116.

33. Read more about why feathers and Psalm 91:4 meant so much to Carollynn at http://www.featherfund.org /the_story.htm.

34. 2 Corinthians 5:7, NIV

35. 2 Corinthians 5:7

36. Excerpted from a 2001 devotional, "God Keeps His Promises," on Dave and Jan Dravecky's Outreach of Hope ministry website (renamed Endurance with Jan and Dave Dravecky). Although this devotional is no longer available, you can find many other resources at http://www.endurance.org.

37. John Piper, "Don't Waste Your Cancer," DesiringGod .org, February 15, 2006, http://www.desiringgod.org /resource-library/taste-see-articles/dont-waste-your-cancer.

About the Author

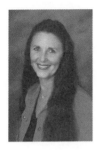

Lynn Eib is a long-time cancer survivor, journalist, and patient advocate, who has provided emotional and spiritual support to tens of thousands of cancer patients and their caregivers. The Cancer Prayer Support Group she founded in 1991 and still facilitates is believed to be the country's longest-running such faith-based group.

She is the author of the Tyndale best-seller *When God & Cancer Meet*, as well as *Finding the Light in Cancer's Shadow* and *When God & Grief Meet*. Lynn also wrote the inspirational commentary for the *He Cares New Testament with Psalms & Proverbs*, designed for those dealing with serious or chronic illness.

She speaks throughout the country on the topic of integrating faith and medicine and conducts inspiring seminars for people on an unwanted journey with cancer. Since 1996 she has worked as a patient advocate in her oncologist's office, where she also provides genetic counseling for those trying to discover if they have a hereditary cancer-causing mutation.

Lynn loves to encourage the discouraged and firmly believes that laughter is healing medicine. All of her support group meetings start with jokes and end with prayers. For resources and information, visit her website, www.lynneib.com.

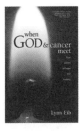
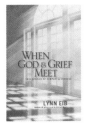
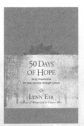
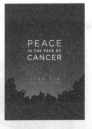